The New Injection Treatment for Impotence

Medical and Psychological Aspects

The New Injection Treatment for Impotence

Medical and Psychological Aspects

Gorm Wagner, M.D., Ph.D.

Helen Singer Kaplan, M.D., Ph.D.

BRUNNER/MAZEL, *Publishers* • NEW YORK

Library of Congress Cataloging-in-Publication Data
Wagner, Gorm.
  The new injection treatment for impotence : medical and
psychological aspects / Gorm Wagner, Helen Singer Kaplan.
     p. cm.
  Includes bibliographical references and index.
  ISBN 0-87630-689-X
  1. Impotence—Chemotherapy.   I. Kaplan, Helen Singer
II. Title.
  [DNLM: 1. Impotence—drug therapy.   2. Injections. WJ 709 W133n]
RC889.W245   1993
616.6'092061—dc20
DNLM/DCL
for Library of Congress   92-49232
                                                                    CIP

Published by
BRUNNER/MAZEL, INC.
19 Union Square West
New York, New York 10003

Manufactured in the United States of America

10 9 8 7 6 5 4 3 2 1

Dedicated to

Helle and Charles

our long suffering spouses
whose vacations were spoiled
by this book

Contents

Preface

We intend this book to supply professionals who take care of men and couples with sexual problems with accurate, up to date, in depth, technical information about the new intracavernosal injection treatment for impotence (ICI), along with practical suggestions and guidelines for the appropriate and effective medical and psychiatric use of this new technology.

We expect that increasing numbers of patients will be asking their doctors and therapists about this "state-of-the-art" treatment and we hope that the material presented in this volume will serve to clarify, demystify, and depoliticize this latest development in sexual medicine.

We further hope that this book will call attention to recent advances in impotence research and to the expanding field of sexual medicine. This much neglected area of health care deserves more attention both in clinical practice and in medical school curricula.

Finally, we hope that the multidisciplinary authorship of this book will underscore the concept that sexual disorders are multifactorial and involve the interface of established disciplines like physiology, andrology, urology, gynecology, psychology, endocrinology, neurology, psychiatry, pharmacology, internal medicine, and general surgery. Only through a concerted effort of many professionals who are expert in these specialties will it be possible to establish sufficient scientific information so that the new generations of medical doctors and other health professionals, unlike so many of their predecessors, will be comfortable and knowledgable about treating human sexual misery.

The areas of expertise of the two authors are sharply demarcated. As indicated in the Table of Contents, we have each written different sections, except for Chapter I which represents a joint effort. GW is responsible for the chapters on the biological basis and medical management of ICI, while HSK has described the psychiatric aspects of this treatment and its consequences in terms of the patient's sexual life.

GORM WAGNER
HELEN SINGER KAPLAN

CHAPTER **I**

Historical Perspectives

by Helen Singer Kaplan
& Gorm Wagner

A. The History of Modern Sexology

by Helen Singer Kaplan

RECENT DECADES have witnessed dramatic advances in our understanding of the mechanisms of erection and in our ability to treat impotence. Until very recently, remarkably little was known about the physiology of the human sexual response or about sexual pathology. Thus, in the sixties our concepts about the etiology of sexual disorders were still completely erroneous and treatment was so ineffective that many patients who suffer from what we now think of as minor erection difficulties were doomed to a lifetime of chronic impotence.

This appalling situation did not come about because sexuality is especially complicated. In fact, sexology is basically much simpler than, for example, neurology or cardiology, which were far more advanced. But sexual medicine lagged far behind the rest of medicine because the puritanical attitudes prevailing in our society until the advent of the "sexual revolution" had made the scientific study of human sexuality impossible until just a few years ago.

Actually, interest in the treatment of impotence dates

back to the very beginnings of medicine. Pre-Christian societies were unabashedly interested in sex and placed great importance on sexual adequacy. Thus, it is not surprising that the writings of such distinguished Greco-Roman physicians and philosophers as Hippocrates, Lucretius and Pliny the Elder contain extensive discussions of remedies for impotence and infertility.

Despite this promising beginning, because of the singular moralistic significance ascribed to human sexual behavior in the Judeo-Christian dogma, sexology was the last of the biological disciplines to cast off the shackles that had hampered medical research in the Western world for some two thousand years. And so, while the other specialities were rapidly advancing into the nuclear age, sexual medicine had, until recently, remained in the dark ages.*

Today, the situation is completely different. Thanks to the amazing progress made since the scientific study of human sexuality became socially acceptable during the forties, we now have a clear understanding of the human sexual response and of the pathogenesis of sexual disorders. As a result, the modern multidisciplinary approach to the treatment of sexual disorders has become so effective that we can now help the majority of patients with potency problems.

---

*The work of the Dutch physician de Graaf, who studied the mechanism of penile erection and circulation using cadavers over 300 years ago, is an exception.

THE SCIENTIFIC STUDY OF SEX

The Pioneering Work of Masters and Johnson

The first significant breakthrough that ushered in the modern era of clinical sexology was made by William H. Masters and Virginia E. Johnson. Their great contribution actually consisted of a rather simple study, but one that would have been unthinkable in the old antisexual days. With scientific objectivity, these two courageous scientists painstakingly observed and recorded 14,000 separate human sexual acts. In their laboratory, behind a one-way mirror, they watched men and women masturbate, engage in intercourse in various positions, have oral sex, have anal sex, have sex while the woman was menstruating, and so on.

Masters and Johnson documented the human sexual response with the help of special recording devices. For example, they developed a method for attaching electrodes to, and recording the muscle activity of, the genitalia during intercourse. They built a camera into a translucent plastic phallus and used this to record vaginal responses during sexual stimulation. In their landmark book, *The Human Sexual Response*, which was published in 1966, Masters and Johnson finally gave the world a carefully documented, accurate, scientific description of the physiology of the male and the female sex organs.

But this descriptive analysis of genital functioning, although extremely useful, was only a first step. The next great breakthrough was the reconceptualization of the outdated monistic view of human sexuality. A new triphasic paradigm corrected some of the old erroneous views of sexual physiology and of the pathogenesis of sexual disorders, while also incorporating the motivational aspects of sex into the model of human sexuality (Kaplan, 1977, 1979).

The Triphasic Concept of Human Sexuality and the Sexual Disorders

Since the beginning of time, the human sexual response had been considered to be a single physiological entity, commencing with arousal, developing into excitement, and ending in a climax. This was a major error that gave rise to another serious misconception: that all sexual disorders were variants of a single clinical entity that was labeled "impotence" in men and "frigidity" in women.

We now know that in actual fact the human sexual response of males and females is composed of three related, but neurophysiologically and anatomically distinct phases: *sexual desire, sexual excitement* and *orgasm*, and we have learned that there are a number of different, clinically distinct sexual disorders that require different treatment approaches.

The first step in dispelling the myth that all sexual disorders were simply forms of impotence or frigidity was made by James Semans, a urologist, before Masters and Johnson's work was published. In a short paper, Semans described the successful treatment of eight premature ejaculators by a procedure now known as the "stop-start" method of interrupted penile stimulation (Semans, 1956). Prior to Semans' astute clinical observations, premature ejaculation (PE) had been classified and treated (unsuccessfully) as a form of impotence, which was then termed "ejaculatory impotence."

The true significance of Semans' discovery was not realized for a long time. But in retrospect we now know that apart from inventing an ingenious method for treating PE, which is still, with some modifications, used today (Kaplan, 1989a), Semans was the first to distinguish between erectile failure or impotence, and PE, which is a failure of ejaculatory control but does not involve erection difficulties.*

The last chapter in the evolution of the modern concept of sexual disorders came in the late seventies as a result of reviewing our treatment failures. By then, we had advanced to a "biphasic" view of sexuality, which recognized the clinical distinction between and the different treatment requirements of erectile and ejaculatory disorders; sex therapy had been developed to a point where it was so effective that any treatment failure warranted a closer look. The analysis of our failures led to the realization that some male patients who had complained of impotence had not improved because we had made an error in our assessment. We had treated these patients with our standard sex therapy protocol for impotence because we had not recognized that their complaints of erectile failure had been secondary to their diminished sexual interest, and that they were actually suffering from *low (hypoactive) sexual desire*** (Kaplan, 1977, 1979). These patients had attempted to make love to their wives out of a sense of duty although they felt little desire. Not surpris-

---

*In 1974, I drew an analogous distinction between female anorgasmia and inhibited female excitement (Kaplan, 1974b). Prior to this, female excitement and orgasm disorders had been subsumed under the single wastebasket term, "frigidity" and this confusion had similarly resulted in poor treatment outcomes.

**Hypo-active* sexual desire (HSD) is the preferred term when the etiology of a patient's deficient sexual desire is not known. By contrast, *inhibited* sexual desire (ISD) specifically designates low-desire states that have only psychological and no physical causes.

ingly, they had developed problems in attaining and maintaining their erections.

One reason for our oversight was that these men had found it less threatening to their partners to complain about their own performance problems than to admit to having lost their sexual interest in their partners. In our desire to support the couples' relationships, we had "bought into" their denial. Once we became aware of this, we found that the complaints of many of our impotent patients centered around dissatisfaction with the subjective aspects of sex—lust or desire.

We now know that desire is an important aspect of human sexuality and that inhibited sexual desire is a distinct psychosexual disorder. Moreover, patients with deficient sexual desire have a poor response to sex therapy methods that are designed for treating psychogenic impotence, although they do well with other forms of sex therapy.

The separation of the sexual disorders into the different phase-related syndromes has had significant clinical implications.* The triphasic system of classification provides the theoretical basis for understanding the distinctive clinical features as well as the pathogenesis of impotence, as distinct from sexual problems of desire or ejaculation. Ultimately, these insights have led to the development of specific and more effective treatments for impotence, as well as for the other sexual disorders.

---

*The human sexual response can actually be divided into four physiologically discrete phases: desire, excitement, orgasm, and resolution. The term Resolution was used by Masters and Johnson to designate the return of the genitalia to their quiescent phase. But the commonly used nosology is *triphasic* rather than the more awkward *quadrophasic* because impairments of orgasm (retarded and premature ejaculation), excitement (Impotence), and desire (HD, ISD, and Sexual Aversion) are common, while clinical disorders of the resolution phase are extremely rare (Kaplan, 1992).

TABLE I.1

The Three Phases of the Male Sexual Response Cycle

Phase	Physiology	Syndromes
I Desire	Activation of CNS sex-regulatory centers; Testosterone required	1. HSD 2. Sexual aversion Impotence
II Excitement (Penile Erection)	1. Penile blood vessels dilate, increasing inflow 2. Smooth muscles relax, blocking outflow	
III Orgasm (Ejaculation)	1. *Emission:* smooth muscles contract collecting semen in posterior urethra 2. *Ejection:* rhythmic contractions of striated IC & BC muscles propel semen out of the urethral meatus.	1. Premature ejaculation 2. Retarded ejaculation

According to the triphasic concept of Human Sexuality (Table I.1) the sexual response of males (and females) is composed of: one, *sexual desire*, which represents the subjective experience of lust that accompanies the activation of the sex regulatory centers in the limbic brain; two, *sexual excitement*, which is a local vasocongestive response that changes the male genitalia from their quiescent state to the erect reproductive phallus; and three, the *orgasm* phase, which in males consists of two subphases—*emission* and *ejection*, which are produced by the reflexive contractions of smooth and striated genital muscles respectively.

THE CLINICAL FEATURES OF THE MALE SEXUAL DISORDERS

Under nonpathological circumstances, sexual desire, excitement, and orgasm overlap in time. This, along with the synchrony that normally exists between the three phases of the sexual response cycle, makes it appear as a single, smooth sequence. But the essential biological discreteness of libido, erection, and ejaculation is clearly revealed in pathological states. For the male, sexual response is seldom destroyed completely, either by organic disease or by psychological stressors. In clinical practice, we typically see the impairment of one of the three phases, while the others are spared. The clinical features of the various sexual dysfunction syndromes are the results of this phase-specific pattern of impairment (Kaplan, 1977, 1979). (See Table I.1)

The chief clinical feature of *impotence* is the failure to attain or maintain an erection firm enough for vaginal intercourse. However, impotent men often retain their interest in sex and many can experience pleasurable ejaculations although their penis remains flaccid. It is only the erectile or vasocongestive excitement phase of the sexual response cycle that is impaired in impotence.

On the other hand, men with *retarded or premature ejaculation* (RE or PE) generally have normal sexual desire and, unless they develop secondary impotence, have no erectile difficulties. These patients suffer from *overcontrol* of the ejaculatory reflex, which is the chief clinical feature of retarded ejaculation, or from *inadequate control*, which characterizes premature ejaculation.

Men with *hypoactive sexual desire* have no primary potency or ejaculatory disorders. The diagnostic criterion for HSD is a lack of sexual desire, which may be global or confined to the partner. Unless secondary impotence complicates the clinical picture, these patients are capable of having intercourse, albeit mechanically and without much pleasure.

The different sexual syndromes are produced by different sets of causes and they respond to different treatment strategies. *The clinical significance of this concept extends to ICI, in that this is an appropriate treatment modality only for erectile difficulties and should be used exclusively to treat impotence. This therapy is of questionable value, and in some cases is potentially harmful for patients with ejaculatory and desire phase sexual disorders.*

SEX THERAPY

Before Masters and Johnson published their groundbreaking volume, "Human Sexual Inadequacy" (1970), it was believed that psychosexual disorders are always the product of severe unconscious neurotic sexual conflicts that originate in serious childhood trauma. In accordance with this theory, lengthy and costly psychoanalytic treatment was recommended for every impotent patient. But the results were extremely poor.

Masters and Johnson made their second immensely important contribution by demonstrating that the psychoanalytic formulation of psychosexual symptoms was not necessarily valid in all cases and that extensive insight therapy was not the best treatment for the majority of patients with sexual dysfunctions. They found that in many cases psychogenic sexual disabilities are the product of less complex and more consciously recognized causes, such as the simple fear of not being able to perform sexually.

Moreover, they demonstrated that long-standing sexual problems, such as impotence and PE, could often be cured rapidly, in two weeks, with their highly innovative cognitive–behavioral, couples oriented therapy program, which stresses the reduction of performance anxiety and improvement of the partners' communications. Masters and Johnson published the results of their remarkably successful rapid treatment program in 1970, and some people thought this spelled the end of psychoanalysis.

But this did not happen. It turned out that a significant proportion of sexually dysfunctional individuals, as well as their partners, are resistant to the rapid behavioral modification of their sexual symptoms because of their concurrent deeper emotional, sexual, and/or marital conflicts. Thus, in the seventies, in order to meet the challenge of the resistant patient, a new sex therapy approach was developed that combines the behavioral modification of sexual symptoms of classic sex therapy with brief, active, psychodynamically oriented management of the patient's resistances (Kaplan, 1974a). This integrated approach, called "The New Sex Therapy," has been widely accepted.

The New Sex Therapy

Brief, psychodynamically oriented sex therapy employs structured erotic interactions that the couple or patient carry out in the privacy of their home. These therapeutic behavioral interventions, which include but are not limited to those invented by Masters and Johnson, are designed to modify such "immediate" psychological causes of the patient's sexual dysfunctions as sexual performance anxiety, partner pressure, and negative self-observations. The therapeutic "homework assignments" are integrated with office sessions, usually on a weekly basis. These are devoted to the psychodynamically oriented exploration of the couple's deeper emotional and relationship problems, to the extent this is necessary, and, most importantly, to the brief, active management of any resistances that may arise (on the part of either partner) to the rapid behavioral modification of the patient's impotence (Kaplan, 1974, 1979, 1987, 1992).

The vast clinical experience accumulated over the past 25 years, and respected by many talented sex therapists, has yielded an accurate understanding of the pathogenesis of impotence and has spawned the development of sophisticated and effective techniques for the rapid modification of sexual symptoms, and for the management of patient resistance, which is a major issue in sex therapy.

These sex therapy concepts and techniques have important applications for dealing with the universally pervasive problem of noncompliance to ICI (see Chapter VI).

ADVANCES IN SEXUAL MEDICINE

In the eighties came a surge of medical advances. Now that sex had become a legitimate subject of scientific inquiry, laboratories all over the world were actively investigating the physiology and biochemistry of erection, orgasm, and sexual desire. This led to an increased understanding of the *mechanisms of erection* and the *physiopathogenesis of impotence* (see Chapter II). The new multidisciplinary efforts also opened the way for the development of new diagnostic (see Chapter III) and treatment methods (see Chapter IV) that are changing the practice of sexual medicine.

The New Diagnostic Methods

Among these are portable NPT monitors for home use, penile doppler circulation studies that could be done as an office procedure, sophisticated radiologic methods for assessing penile bloodflow and anatomy more accurately, genital neurophysiologic tests, and simple blood tests that can reliably measure sex hormones with great accuracy. These became available in the eighties and are now used routinely to evaluate impotent patients prior to beginning treatment. Current methods of the assessment of impotence are described in detail in Chapter II.

This new technology has allowed clinicians to detect subtle physical problems that had previously been missed and also to assess the extent of physical impairments with greater accuracy. The data accumulated with the help of these new diagnostic methods have made it clear that physical determinants are far more prevalent in the etiology of potency problems than had previously been believed. In the past, it had been thought that impotence was predominantly a psychogenic disorder, with organic factors accounting for as little as five percent of erectile complaints. While this has proven to be true for younger patients, we now know that at least 50 percent of impotent men who are over 50 years of age have some disease state that affects their sexual organs, or are taking medications with sexual side effects, or have demonstrable and advanced presbyrectic physical changes (Kaplan, 1989b). It goes without saying that psychological treatment is ineffective for men whose impotence is exclusively or mostly organic, but in many cases patients with physical problems are excellent candidates for ICI.

Treatment of Older Patients

There is convincing evidence that sex remains important to many people into advanced old age. For this reason, the potency problems of older men should not be neglected. Injection therapy is of great value for treating older men with impotence of organic and mixed (physical and psychological) etiology. Chapter VII is devoted to this topic.

The New Physical Treatments

The eighties saw the development of numbers of innovative new medical treatments for impotence. In addition to the new injection treatment for impotence, which we consider to be the most important development of the eighties in sexual medicine, these include improved methods of penile implant surgery, new procedures in vascular surgery, more sophisticated hormone treatments for men with endocrine problems, and some new drug approaches to the treatment of sexual dysfunctions.

Medication

Two types of medications are currently used in the treatment of impotence: psychoactive drugs, which aim to improve sexual functioning by lowering sexual anxiety or by relieving depression, and substances that exert stimulating effects on the genitalia or on the sex regulatory mechanisms of the brain.

Antianxiety medications such as aprezolam (Xanax) do not improve potency directly. These substances affect sexuality in a positive direction by improving the patient's emotional state. More specifically, excellent antianxiety agents are available that can be valuable adjuvants in the therapy of impotent patients with severe and intractable performance anxiety. Adjuvant medication that blocks panic attacks, such as Desyrel (trazodone), is particularly effective for impotent patients with concurrent panic disorders, who are frequently too anxious to be able to cooperate with or benefit from sex therapy unless they are medicated (Kaplan, 1982, 1987).

While *Depression* has no direct deleterious effects on penile erection, depressed men often lose their libido and may develop secondary potency difficulties on that account. When a patient has little interest in sex or in living because he feels sad, management of the depression, often with the aid of antidepressant medications, is indicated prior to instituting sex therapy or ICI. For it makes little sense, nor is it usually effective, to attempt to override or bypass the patient's depression and lack of sexual desire with pharmacologically induced erections.

The use of psychopharmacologic agents for men with erectile dysfunctions requires considerable experience and expertise in sexual medicine. That is because many antianxiety and antidepressant agents also have sexual side effects and interfere with erection or ejaculation or libido on a physical basis (Klein, 1987; Segraves, 1988, 1992). The clinician must choose agents with low profiles of sexual side effects, e.g. Desyrel (trazodone), Eldepril (depronil), or Wellbutrin (buproprion), and he or she must titrate the doses very carefully, aiming at the "therapeutic window"—a dose high enough to relieve the patient's dysphoria, but low enough to avoid creating drug-induced sexual impairments.

Sexual Stimulants

After millennia of searching in vain for the holy Grail of sexually stimulating potions, we are finally reaching the age of true aphrodisiacs. Now that the mysteries of the neurophysiology and biochemistry of sexual desire and penile erection are yielding to scientific inquiry, we are beginning to see the development of medications that can improve libido and potency on a chemical basis; at last we can abandon the legendary rhinoceros horns and cantherides.

One substance that has been clinically available for some time is yohimbine (Yokon). In good responders, this drug acts on the penis in a way that favors erections. However, Yohimbine is of limited value in that it is effective in only a small proportion of impotent patients. Moreover, this drug should not be used for patients with underlying anxiety disorders, because it is related to hallucinogenic agents and can precipitate panic attacks in susceptible individuals.

A more promising development lies in drugs that stimulate the sex centers of the brain directly to enhance libido and erections. The first drug in this category to be marketed in the U.S., Wellbutrin (buproprion), was originally developed as an antidepressant (Crenshaw, Goldberg & Stern, 1987). This drug is by no means ideal, because it improves libido significantly in only a minority of patients and there can be unpleasant side effects. However, many other promising medications that may create aphrodisiac effects by manipulating the neurotransmittors that inhibit and activate the CNS sex-regulating centers are on the drawing board. Hopefully, we will soon have new and more effective medical treatments for impotence and deficient sexual desire states.

B.   The Development of Injection Therapy

by Gorm Wagner

THE MODERN DEVELOPMENT of medical methods for reinstating a normal function of the penis in men who suffered from erectile dysfunction was initiated by the Czech vascular surgeon Vaclav Michal (1973). In the early 1970's he developed a surgical technique to revascularize the erectile tissue of the cavernous body.

After his first publications, several European surgeons visited Prague to watch his technique. One requirement for good results in this type of surgery was a proper preoperative selection of the right candidates. This was done by a procedure called phallo-arteriography. An injection of radio-contrast medium in the arterial tree at the point where the pudendal artery branches off from the iliac artery was given to visualize the arteries on a series of X-rays.

At the same time, normal saline was infused directly into the cavernous bodies to produce an increase of volume and to stretch the structures inside the penis to optimize the quality of the investigation. Sometimes papaverine was injected into the arteries to prevent them from closing off, a simple procedure commonly used by vascular surgeons during surgery.

After some years, the procedures of Michal attracted the attention of a French radiologist, Ginestié (1976), who refined the technique of selective pudendal arteriography. Other vascular surgeons looked into this possible new treatment of "arteriogenic" impotence and started to revascularize.

Simultaneously, other developments occurred. The Danish surgeon Jørgen Ebbehøj (1975) had developed a new and very simple technique to treat priapism (long-standing erection, which passes through a painful stage into destruction of the internal trabecular structures of cavernous bodies, leaving a fibrous and unfunctional organ if the condition has lasted for 12 hours or longer). By a small incision through the glans, he let the knife cut an opening between the rigid and stiff cavernous body and the unaffected and flaccid spongious body, enabling the trapped blood to escape into the spongious body and drain back to the venous system. The priapism then disappeared (Ebbehøj, 1975). However, those who continued to have an open leak during the months following surgery were not able to regain their ability to erect. Others in whom the surgically induced opening had closed did not have erectile problems. This could be studied through cavernosography, which is infusion of contrast medium into the cavernous body to visualize where it may leak. A simple surgical closure of the leak brought back normal erection.

When in 1975 a young man of 17 years with primary erectile dysfunction was referred to Ebbehøj, he performed a cavernosography and found a large leak. This was surgically closed and the man was able to erect normally. This led us to study those men referred for erectile problems. A standardized penile infusion technique was developed that at the same time was followed by visual sexual stimulation, sometimes enabling us to demonstrate an abnormal drainage at the moment when a normal erection should have occurred. Instead the blood of the cavernous bodies started escaping (Ebbehøj, Uhrenholt & Wagner, 1980).

The developments in Prague and Copenhagen were independent and so was a similar interest of the Rumanian urologist, Tudoriou, who had performed many anatomical studies of the penis, including, on one occasion, a very careful dissection of a young man who had committed suicide, leaving a note saying he had done so because of his inability to have a normal erection. During that autopsy, a large (congenital) opening through the tunica albuginea was demonstrated, clearly indicating an anatomical defect similar to the ones found in Copenhagen by cavernosography, and surgically correctable (Ebbehøj & Wagner, 1979; Tudorio & Bourmer, 1983).

During the same period in the mid 1970s it also became clear to some physiological investigators that the nervous control of erection in man was not clearly understood. The neurotransmission between the nerves and the smooth muscles of the arteries and the trabecular tissue was believed to be cholinergic, which meant, for instance, that atropine, which blocks the function of acetylcholine, would prevent erection through transmission blockade. An animal study in England of baboons had shown that erection provoked by stimulation through electrodes on sacral nerves was not prevented by atropine infusion (Brindley & Craggs, 1975). My reaction to this was that this experiment could easily be conducted in man.

One evening in the fall of 1977 I called a colleague and

asked him to give me an intravenous atropine injection since I wanted to study the effect of atropine on sexual performance. Reluctantly, he agreed. I got my i.v. in his kitchen, with my wife in the car outside with the motor running. The usual signs of atropinization, like increase of heart rate, blurred vision, and dry mouth, appeared. After a fast return to our house, a completely normal sexual performance with erection and orgasm, but with all the signs of atropine effect still present, was achievable.

A month later in London, I met with the British physiologist, Giles Brindley, who had performed the experiments on the baboons. We discussed the mysterious neurotransmission of erection and I told him about my experiment. He too, had taken atropine and had found that it did not prevent erection.

We felt we were on an interesting track and agreed to do a study together. In early 1978 Brindley came to my lab in Copenhagen. A group of men who were able to have normal erections volunteered to participate in a study where ordinary registered drugs would be given to them in doses used clinically.

The result of the atropine study was clear-cut after we had established that they could erect normally on stimuli like penile vibration and visual sexual stimulation and could repeat this during full atropinization. Another drug, propranolol, a β blocking agent used to treat arterial hypertension, was tried next and in none of the participants did it affect normal sexual performance at home or erection in the lab.

The third compound we tried was oral intake of phenoxybenzamine. Even at fairly large doses it did not prevent erection. However, it completely abolished ejaculation due to the α-adrenergic blockade of the ejaculatory ducts. One peculiar observation was made: The penis had considerably changed in size to a larger and more voluminous organ, an effect that lasted 20-30 hours after oral intake. Erection was very easily obtained, but not at a level that could be detected as different from the situations with no drug (Wagner & Brindley, 1980).

The work of Michal had spread to the east coast of the United States and the American urologist, Adrian Zorginiotti, summoned a two day meeting in New York City in September of 1978. Around 100 participated on a gray Saturday; only a handful were from Europe. That meeting became the turning point, changing forever the old, erroneous way of thinking of impotence as being exclusively a psychogenic problem. New findings and surprising presentations of new ideas and possibilities were discussed. Another meeting was scheduled for 1980 in Monaco, to be followed by Copenhagen in 1982. Thus, a group of clinicians and researchers interested in erection and impotence was gradually shaped and finally developed into the International Society of Impotence Research.

The focus of this group was mainly on developing new diagnostic tests and on substantiating and accepting the theory of abnormal drainage. New surgical approaches, not least by the French vascular surgeon, Ronald Virag, were tried out.

In the summer of 1978, a paper had been published by a pharmacology group from New Orleans describing experiments on cats to study the effect of the sympathetic nervous system upon the bladder function; observations on erection were also included (Domer et al., 1978).

Unfortunately, as often happens in scientific publications, the paper passed without much attention. It demonstrated very clearly that if the alpha-blocking agent phentolamine was injected in (fairly) large doses, penile erection occurred. The authors concluded that adrenergic innervation of the penis was what kept it flaccid and that this state could be changed into erection by the blocking of the adrenergic tone.

Back in Copenhagen, a young Ph.D. student, Bent Ottesen, who worked in my lab suggested that vasoactive intestinal polypeptide (VIP) might be a candidate of interest in the neurotransmission leading to erection. He had shown the abundance of VIP in the female reproductive organs and a series of possible functional roles of this recently discovered signal-peptide. We shifted interest and conducted studies on the male organs and VIP, Some of these were done together with Virag in Paris. It became clear that VIP was present in the trabecular tissue of the penis, that it relaxed the smooth muscle, and that it could be detected in affluent blood from the penis during erection (Willis et al., 1981; Ottesen et al., 1984).

At the Monaco meeting in 1980, both Michal and Virag could report on patients who after only one artificial erection with saline had experienced a significant improvement of their erection. This was discussed at length at the meeting, but nobody could give a clue to the mechanism underlying this experience. Generally, it was believed that it might be due to psychological factors because the patient himself now had seen his own penis being erect. Both investigators refused the theory as they had observed that patients under full anesthesia also had reported the improvement of erections.

One day in June of 1982 in Paris, where we were conducting some new diagnostic investigations, Virag told me about an observation he had made. During a surgical procedure when he was going to free the epigastric inferior artery, he erroneously had injected papaverine into a vessel leading into the penis instead of into the epigastric artery. The infusion resulted in a rigid erection of two hours duration. This observation made him think that papaverine could induce erection and that it might be beneficial in situations of artificial erections that were normally done with saline infusion into the cavernous body.

Because of his observation of the effects of papaverine, Virag did two investigations: One with 15 patients diagnosed as arteriogenic and 10 diagnosed as nonorganic. They all had an 80 mg papaverine injection intracavernosally and were closely monitored for two hours. Fifty percent of the organic and none of the nonorganic experienced improved erection.

Another group of 30 patients with arteriogen etiology (including 12 diabetics) had 80 mg of papaverine injected intracavernosally and this was followed 15 minutes later by a normal saline infusion into the penis. The procedure was repeated two months later. Four patients became normally functional, nine improved significantly, and one had no change of erectile capacity.

I urged Virag to present these findings and open them up for discussion at the meeting two months later in Copenhagen. He preferred, however, not to have his new findings discussed, but decided to have them published quickly as a letter to the editor in the prestigious British medical journal, *The Lancet* (Figure I.1) (Virag, 1982). During the discussion, he also told about a colleague who had used papaverine by self-injection and experienced two episodes of prolonged erection that had to be attended to. Virag expressed concern about what might happen if this type of self-therapy became widespread because of the potential for abuse.

Shortly before the meeting in August, 1982 in Copenhagen, Brindley announced that due to intense research activity he did not have the time to participate. However, the meeting went very well and some American groups reported on having identified new groups of patients who developed a iatrogenic erectile dysfunction as a result of prostatic treatment and others who realized the abnormal drainage factor as being a substantial factor in many cases of impotence.

Behind the scene was the undisclosed knowledge of Virag, the unknown "research activity" of Brindley, and, even more interesting, the lack of notice to anyone that an American general practitioner, Latorre, from El Paso, Texas had patented in 1978 a double-barreled syringe to be used for penile intracavernosal injection of vasoactive compounds to produce erection, although he never suggested which drug or what dose (U.S., Patent 4, 127, 118).

On his way back to France, Virag posted his letter-to-the-editor before he left Denmark and it was published in *The Lancet* on October 23, 1982.

The research of Brindley turned out to be experiments of injection of alpha-blocking agents in patients who were unable to achieve erection. Some of these patients were paraplegic, while others were completely unable to have an erection. He taught the patients or their wives how to inject, using phenoxybenzamine after he had tried and discarded phentolamine as being unable to produce a full erection. Thus, the first self-injection program was developed.

This report was presented by Brindley at a meeting of

INTRACAVERNOUS INJECTION OF PAPAVERINE FOR ERECTILE FAILURE

Sir,—The mechanism for the filling of the cavernous bodies at the onset of erection is still in dispute.[1] Accidental intracavernous injection of papaverine during a surgical shunting procedure[2] produced a prolonged fully rigid erection of two hours' duration. This fact, combined with observation of improvement of erectile function reported by impotent patients after they had been subjected to artificial erection[3] for evaluation of erectile dysfunction,[4] led us to study the effect of intracavernous injection of papaverine.

The study was done after the thorough investigations (including nocturnal penile tumescence monitoring, pudendal arteriography, and bulbocavernous reflex latency measurements) that we recommend for evaluation of erectile dysfunction.[3,4] In this way we could classify cases as organic or non-organic impotence.

80 mg papaverine was injected into one of the cavernous bodies, after insertion into the other of a 21G plastic needle for continuous monitoring of intracavernous pressure (ICP). To study the condition of arterial vessels, ultrasonic continuous measurement (Doppler method) and pulse plethysmography were used. Later, selective bilateral internal iliac arteriography was done. Our preliminary findings relate to fifteen organic cases and ten non-organic cases of impotence.

The immediate reaction was an increase in ICP, indicating volume charges and the development of pressure inside the cavernous bodies. The mean value of the ICP increase was much higher when the trial was done during general anaesthesia (mean ICP increase 70 mm Hg compared with 40 mm Hg without anaesthesia). This effect was related to increased arterial flow, as shown by Doppler studies, plethysmography, and arteriography. The peak effect, depending on the state of the arteries, was obtained after 2–15 min, and an effect lasted for from 10 to 120 min. There were no general or local complications.

Seven of the fifteen patients with an organic aetiology reported significantly improved erections in the days after the procedure but none of the non-organic cases reported any changes in their erectile capability. All seven had arterial lesions in the distral part of the internal pudendal artery and/or in the cavernous arteries.

In the light of these results thirty impotent patients (including twelve with diabetes mellitus) who had Doppler and arteriographic evidence of arterial insufficiency were selected for conservative therapy. Intracavernous injection of papaverine (80 mg) was followed, after 15 min observation of the drug's effect, by infusion of 1% heparin in normal saline via an infusion pump, to obtain and maintain a rigid erection for a 15 min period. No anaesthesia was used.

The procedure was repeated 2 months later and then every third month or according to the clinical status. Of the fourteen patients (seven with diabetes) who had two or more artificial erections, four reported a return to a normal sexual life; nine described a significant improvement in penile rigidity; in one there was no effect and an arterial revascularisation procedure was done.

Few clinical studies have been done on the effects of drugs on penile erection.[5] No vasoactive drug has proved effective in controlled studies. Papaverine is a powerful smooth-muscle relaxant and has been used in laboratory studies of vasoactive drugs, as a control substance.[6] Two levels of action seem possible: inhibition of cyclic AMP phosphodiesterase[7] or an antinicotinic effect.[8] Artificial erections achieved with normal saline are associated with vasodilatation of branches of the pudendal arteries,[9] and we agree that there must be mechanical action at the level of the cavernous tissue.

I thank Dr Gorm Wagner, Panum Institute, University of Copenhagen, for comments.

R. VIRAG

Centre for Study and Research on Impotence
65 bis rue Nicolo,
Paris 75016, France

1. Wagner G, Bro Rasmussen F, Willis EA, Nielsen MH. New theory on the mechanism of erection involving hitherto undescribed vessels. *Lancet* 1982; i; 416–18.
2. Michal V, Kramer R, Pospichal J. Arterial epigastrico cavernous anastomosis for the treatment of sexual impotence. *World J Surg* 1977; 1: 515–20.
3. Virag R, Zwang G, Dermange H, Legman M. Utilisation de l'erection passive dans l'exploration de l'impuissance d'origine vasculaire. *Contracept Fertil Sexual* 1979; 7: 707–10.
4. Virag R, Zwang G, Dermange H, Legman M. Vasculogenic impotence: a review of 92 cases with 54 surgical operations. *Vasc Surg* 1981; 15: 9–17.
5. Wagner G, Green R. Impotence, physiological, psychological and surgical diagnosis and treatment. New York: Plenum Press, 1981.
6. Betz E, Ingvar DH. Regional blood flow in the cerebral cortex measured by heat and inert gas clearence. *Acta Physiol Scand* 1967; 1–9.
7. Posch G, Kukometz WR. Papaervine induced inhibition of phosphodiesterase activity in various mammalian tissues. *Life Sci* 1969; 10: 133–44.
8. Bauer V, Caper R. Studies on the neuropharmacology of papaverine. *Neuropharmacology* 1972; 11: 697–700.
9. Michal V, Pospichal J. Phalloarteriography in the diagnosis of corpus cavernosography. *Radiology* 1976; 119; 69–73.

Figure I.1. Virag's original contribution published in *The Lancet.* (Reprinted with permission from *The Lancet,* October 23, 1982.)

the Physiological Society in Cambridge in April of 1983. The abstract had been submitted in the fall of 1982 without his knowing of the Virag paper. In 1983, a detailed paper by Brindley appeared in the *British Journal of Psychiatry* (Brindley 1983a, b). As a result he was invited to the annual meeting of the American Urological Association in Las Vegas in 1983.

This lecture became an unforgettable milestone in the history of this established professional association. Urologists do not close their eyes to problems of incontinence, foul diseases, or sexual inadequacy. However, none of these subjects had ever been presented so graphically to this group as was done on this occasion by a colleague demonstrating clinically the effects of self-injection.

Brindley had been challenged before the lecture by one of the sponsors who suggested, "Why don't you demonstrate that this works?" As a true researcher, he took this suggestion seriously and injected himself with phenoxybenzamine before the lecture. Then he proceeded to give the lecture and ended it by opening his pants and demonstrating the effect of the injection on his own membrum to the astonished and unprepared audience of urologists, very few of whom had ever experienced the sight of another man's erect penis.

In 1984, the biennial meeting of the International Society for Impotence Research (ISIR) was to be held in Paris. Within this group, there was considerable fear of inviting Brindley as guest speaker, an astonishing demonstration of the need for desensitization even within this professional group in the area of their own specialty. As will be seen later in this volume, phenoxybenzamine turned out to be a drug with problems in this use.

At the 1984 meeting in Paris Zorgniotti presented the

first five patients on self-injection using the combination of papaverine and phentolamine.

At the following meeting in 1986 in Prague, the Japanese urologist, Ishii, presented the erection-producing effect in man of prostaglandin E_1. His trials were based on the results of experimental *in-vitro* studies by Hedlund and Andersson from Sweden.

Since then, much research has been done in different labs around the world to identify compounds that may act specifically on the tissues involved in erection. We are now at a point where effective and safe agents, which can provoke penile erections, are clinically available and being used worldwide. Finally, the pharmaceutical industry, too, has begun to look into the development of suitable new products.

CHAPTER II

Erection and Impotence

by Gorm Wagner

THE PENIS CONSISTS of two corpora cavernosa (the cavernosal bodies), which in the pendular part merge into one
functional unit surrounded by the 2-4 mm thick fibrous
sheet, the tunica albuginea. It is zeppelin shaped and contains a series of internal fibrous strands that serve the purpose of keeping the shaft straight when erect as they run
from side to side as bracing wires.

Underneath the cavernous bodies runs the spongious
body, which contains the urethra and ends with the glans
on the tip of which the urethra opens. The glans covers
and surrounds the end of the cavernous bodies and makes
the termination of the shaft. In circumcised men, the glans
will be free and visible, whereas it usually will be covered
by the foreskin in uncircumcised men. The spongious
body contains a large thick-walled venous network and
cannot achieve the same stiffness (rigidity) as the cavernous
bodies. Thus cavernous and spongious systems are completely separate tissues with different circulatory properties
when it comes to erection.

The main blood flow to the glans comes through two
dorsal arteries that run outside the tunica albuginea in a

small grove closely together with the dorsal nerves and the unpaired deep dorsal vein. The latter drains the glans and spongious body, but also receives blood drained from the cavernous tissue via a system of circumflex veins. Thus, these extra-tunical vessels and nerves function regardless of whether the penis is flaccid or erect, without their function being impaired by tumescence (engorgement of the penis), as they are stretchable.

The cavernous bodies receive their arterial supply through the deep penile artery piercing into each of the crura on their postero-medial surface not far from the area where the crus is closely anchored on its lateral side into the periost of the pelvic bone, which is part of the pelvis.

The artery is followed by the cavernosal nerve, which has just passed through the capsule of the prostate a few millimeters to the side of the prostatic part of the urethra.

If these two nerves are cut, erection cannot occur. Animal experimentation has documented this and shown that immediately after the nerves are severed, there is a slight increase in volume (size) of the penis, followed by a decrease. This alternating situation will continue for hours and gives us a good understanding of the function of the cavernosal nerve, which contains fibers that prevent erection (keep the penis flaccid) and fibers which promote erection when stimulated.

Most likely, the antierectile fibers are from the sympathetic system while the erectile fibers stem from the sacral nerves S_2, S_3, S_4, which as nervi erigentes merge into a complex nerve plexus with fibers from the sympathetic trunk coming through the hypogastric nerve, which contains erectile fibers coming from higher centers in the central nervous system.

Figure II.1 depicts in schematic form this complicated

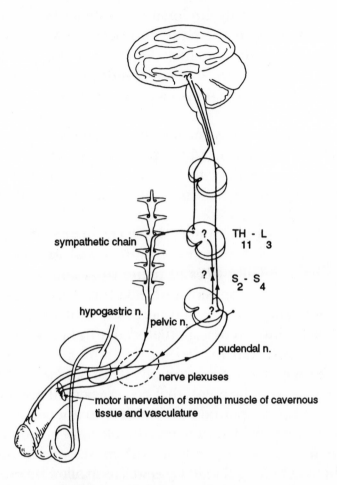

Figure II.1.   Schematic presentation of the nervous system involved in penile erection. Innervation of the penis is from three sources: somatic, sympathetic, and parasympathetic. Somatic sensory fibers run in the pudendal nerve while the motor innervation of the smooth muscles of the vessels and of the tissue of the cavernous bodies derives from the hypogastric nerve and the pelvic nerves (nervi erigentes) forming the nerve plexuses of the pelvis. Besides the innervation shown, other male genital organs receive fibers from the sympathetic and the parasympathetic systems. The question marks indicate the uncertainty of the synaptic transmissions and connections between a sacran and a lumbar center, as well as the cerebral connections in the human. (Wagner & Green, 1981)

and as yet not fully understood system. However, the alternation between increase and decrease in size of the penis in the acute state after denervation also has taught us that there must be a system inside the penis that has an autonomous function once the nervous control has ceased.

When the nerve has entered the cavernous body, it starts branching out, giving fibers partly to the artery and its branches, but mainly to the smooth muscle cell-mass, which is the main constituent of the cavernous body (see Figure II.2).

With the use of laboratory *in-vitro* technique, it has been possible to study the smooth muscle cell in a so-called organ bath. Small pieces of tissue from animals or men can be placed in a physiological solution, kept at constant body-like temperature, and aereated with oxygen, thus being kept alive under simulated natural conditions for many hours (Adaikan, 1979).

In this way, it is possible to study the spontaneous activity of the tissue and the events that occur when different pharmacological compounds are added to the bath. Such studies have provided us with valuable information about the regulation of the penile smooth muscle and its central role in maintaining flaccidity, as well as in allowing erection of the penis to occur.

Through this approach, we have also learned about the role and importance of the naturally occurring neurotransmitters and of the possibilities of interfering with these systems through the action of externally applied pharmacological agents. In addition, direct effects upon the smooth muscles can be studied (Hedlund & Andersson, 1985).

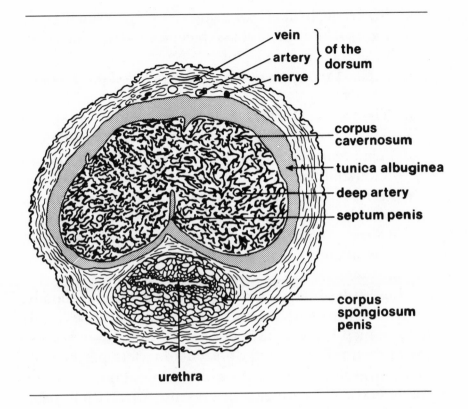

vein ⎫
artery ⎬ of the dorsum
nerve ⎭

corpus cavernosum

tunica albuginea

deep artery

septum penis

corpus spongiosum penis

urethra

Figure II.2. Cross-section of the shaft of the penis. The dominance of the cavernous bodies is shown. The main component of the trabecular tissue is smooth muscle. (Wagner & Green, 1981)

Experiments have established that

1. A certain tone (constant contraction) exists;
2. Spontaneous contractions occur every 1–3 minutes in larger groups of cells;
3. The maintenance and development of further contraction are due to norepinephrine (the sympathetic neurotransmitters). Certain age changes occur in sensitivity to neurotransmitters;

4. Norepinephrine contraction can be prevented by the blocking of alpha-1 receptors with specific receptor-sensitive agents;
5. Alpha-1 receptors dominate over alpha-2 receptors by a factor of 10:1;
6. The cells are able to communicate via gap junctions;
7. The endothelial cells lining the smooth muscle-cells are necessary for the normal function (relaxation and contraction) of the smooth muscle;
8. The substance released from the endothelial cells to induce relaxation is the gas NO. The substance causing contraction is a polypeptide called endothelin.

Thus, such studies have revealed that the penile smooth muscle itself may be altered by age and by disease (local or systemic). This provides a basis for future understanding of such processes and of how to interfere pharmacologically, especially in the possibility of designing specific compounds, and strategies for their use, which could substitute for the loss of naturally occurring agents serving the normal regulation of erection (Hedlund & Andersson, 1985; Wein et al., 1983; Saenz de Tejada et al., 1989; Holmquist et al., 1990; Christ et al., 1990; Wagner, 1991; Rajfer et al., 1992).

As the nervous system locally and centrally is intermingled so closely with the relaxation of penile smooth muscle cells, which is the basic mechanism creating an erection, it is easy to conceive that any change in "normal" neurotransmitter performance may impede the development of erection and that such acute or chronic impairments may be of a basically psychic nature, or age-dependent or disease-dependent.

With our present knowledge, however, we are not able clearly to define the level and/or the principal chemical defaults in a given case.

Only such disorders that can be quantified either visually or by means of quantifiable measures are generally accepted as pathology and, thereby, as a causal factor underlying a symptom of malfunction. It follows, therefore, that malfunctions that are demonstrable only at the level of isolated tissue at this stage of development cannot be used as a diagnostic tool in determination of a cause for a symptom (in this case erectile dysfunction) in an intact human being where scores of external circumstances also may influence the normal function.

Thus, disorders of the neurotransmitters in the brain, spinal cord, or peripheral neural terminals are at this stage beyond our diagnostic capacity.

ARTERIAL SUPPLY

The peripheral arteries and their branches are to a great extent accessible for diagnostic procedures. It is well established that arteriosclerosis of small resistance vessels in the arterial tree is the cause of malfunction locally due to diminished arterial flow regulation that does not enable sufficient flow when demanded. This is a major contributor to impotence. Hypertension, smoking, high blood lipids, and diabetes mellitus are commonly the etiology of these changes, as well as a certain hereditary disposition for arterial disease (Virag et al., 1985).

Originally arterial disease and impotence were linked together by the French surgeon Leriche, who in 1940 noted that a majority of patients with occlusive arterial disorders at the bifurcation of the aorta into the two major arterial trunks of the common iliac arteries suffered from failure of erectile capacity (Leriche, 1940).

It has since been shown that intermittent claudicatio or impotence could be the first sign of arterial occlusive disease of the major arterial trunk. Figure II.3 shows the arterial system that leads to the most important artery in erectile function, the deep penile artery.

By a highly specialized x-ray procedure—the selective pudendal arteriography—it is possible to visualize by infusion of contrast medium the arterial tree serving the penis and thereby to localize the site of an arterial occlusion or the distribution of an arterial lesion that may be the cause of erectile dysfunction.

While the demonstration of an occluded arterial system may be a good indicator of impairment of arterial inflow into the penis, an open system demonstrated during X-ray examination does not necessarily guarantee a normal function (in this case dilatation). During sexual stimulation, an increase in arterial flow is a necessary prerequisite for obtaining a normal erection with sufficient rigidity for vaginal penetration. A certain degree of relaxatory ability of the smooth muscles surrounding the artery and a certain degree of elasticity of the other tissue components are necessary to obtain and to allow maintenance of the necessary increase of diameter of the peripheral arteries to allow the increase in flow and protrusion of the systemic mean arterial pressure into the smaller branches of the penile arterial system (Figure II.3).

The inside of the "resting" (flaccid) cavernous body is characterized of having almost closed spaces with very little content of blood due to the contraction of the cavernous

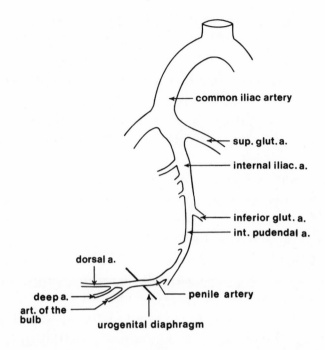

Figure II.3. Schematic presentation of the arterial vessels supplying the penis. (Wagner & Green, 1981)

smooth muscle cells in this state. At the same time, the arteries are well contracted, providing a higher resistance to pressure and perfusion of the penis.

When sexual stimulation occurs, two major events occur in the penis: (1) Dilatation of the arteries and their branches allowing increase of blood flow through the minute openings (helicine end-arteries) into the cavernous spaces, which easily fill up because of decrease of resistance of the cavernosal spaces due to (2) Complete relaxation of the smooth muscles of the cavernosal walls, which are now passively stretched and permit the cavernes to be filled up with blood.

This internal increase of volume and of the resulting pressure impedes the outflow by compressing the subtunical collecting venous system to such an extent that the outflow is reduced, in spite of the pressure gradient. At this moment the pressure inside the cavernous body increases and becomes equal to the mean arterial blood pressure; the increase in arterial inflow then diminishes, or even stops.

In this way, a stable erection is obtained and will be maintained as long as the smooth muscle cells of the arteries and of the cavernous tissue are kept relaxed.

Any event that will increase outflow and/or decrease inflow at this time will destabilize the erection and make the intracavernous pressure fall, leading to insufficient rigidity for vaginal penetration.

From what has been mentioned above, it would seem clear that if the closure mechanism is insufficient it may be possible to obtain sufficiently full erection, but this would be difficult to maintain.

Two major causes exist for defects in the closure mechanism giving rise to abnormal drainage:

1. *Abnormally large veins* can be seen in some patients, where one or several such veins are piercing directly through the tunica albuginea into the venous system. This creates an abnormally high outflow that cannot be stopped by the normal subtunical closure mechanism.

The leakage will not prevent increase in volume (tumescence) of the penis, but as soon as the intracavernosal pressure rises above that of the venous system, the abnormal drainage increases and the developed pressure (rigidity) will drop. If the leaking area is in the pendular, free part of the penis, a rubber band around the root of the penis will prevent the venous backflow and in this way stabilize the erection.

If the leakage is more centrally placed, for instance leading from one or both of the crura, a manual pressure in the perineum behind the scrotum may alleviate the backflow.

Such cases with one or a few well defined large, abnormal veins are obvious candidates for surgical closure of these vessels (Ebbehøj & Wagner, 1979).

2. *Insufficient intracavernosal closure mechanism* is probably the most common cause for abnormal drainage. This is often combined with a slightly reduced capability of dilatation of the penile arteries.

If a reduction of the smooth muscle cell mass has occurred and the tissue instead has been taken over by connective tissue, which has less compliance, the overall function of the trabecular tissue is diminished.

If the environment is cold, the penis will shrink. This will also occur when the man is distressed, frightened, or in any condition where his adrenaline blood level is elevated. On the other hand, in the "resting" phase, that is to say when the temperature is neutral and no sexual stimuli occur, the penis is soft and stretchable (Bondil et al., 1990).

Therefore, when the penis is to be examined by inspection and palpation, which are the two most simple but very important clinical examinations, this has to be done in a quiet atmosphere, in a well-heated room, and uninterrupted by others.

Most men who are seeking help for erection problems

feel uncomfortable once it gets to the examination of the penis. The penis often will shrink in this situation. This gives important information to the examiner as it indicates that the smooth muscles inside the corpora cavernosa are able to be activated, in this case contracted, and that it most likely is under the control of the (autonomous) nervous system and of the CNS.

If the penis at this stage is palpated gently and slightly stretched, the smooth muscles normally "give in" and make a thorough palpation possible. This is a necessary part of the examination as it will be possible to palpate a Peyronie's plaque, which is a hard, cartilage-like area or nodule of fibrotic tissue. In certain cases, a fibrotic area may be the cause of erectile dysfunction, especially if it is linked to the tunica. In such cases, it may prevent the normal shut-off mechanism from functioning, thereby causing abnormal drainage and preventing normal stiffness during sexual arousal.

The stretchability of the flaccid penis is another important factor to observe as it gives an indication of the type of tissue inside the corpus cavernosum. An increase of the proportion of fibrous tissue, which is age-correlated, will decrease the stretchability.

Another indicator of diminished tissue mass is when the shaft is long and thin and the glans looks disproportionately large, making the penis look and feel almost "droopy-tailed" ("Schlappschwanz").

If the patient continues to have a retracted and very firm texture of the shaft, he may very likely have a high degree of anxiety. In other situations, this also may interfere with normal penile function.

The best moment to palpate discrete nodules of fibrosis

is during the first minutes after an intracorporeal injection of a smooth muscle-relaxing agent and before the arteries have opened fully up and the intracavernous spaces start to fill up with blood.

CHAPTER **III**

Pharmacology

by Gorm Wagner

ONCE IT HAD been established that certain pharmacological agents placed inside the cavernous bodies of the penis provoked an erection, the treatment of erectile dysfunction, as well as the diagnostic work-up procedures, changed. However, before the use became widespread, almost no ordinary scientific data on how the drugs were acting locally or on how they were tolerated had been established in larger clinical trials.

The point was that these were well known, older compounds that had been registered and marketed for other purposes. Apparently, no "forced" clinical trials were to be conducted, as the pharmaceutical industry was watching the development from the sidelines only. There seemed to be no hurry as the patents of these drugs were old and the size of the market was not known with any precision.

In most countries, it is the legal right of a physician to prescribe a drug if he/she considers this will benefit the patient.

The drug has to be registered and on the market, but irrespective of the originally approved indications for the registration of the drug, it can be used for any purpose that the physician, in his/her clinical judgment, thinks is desirable. On this basis, clinicians all over the world who saw patients who might benefit from self-injection of papaverine obviously had to seriously consider the prescription of the drug after an individually based evaluation, after testing in the office, indicated that the drug induced an erection and thereby alleviated the patient's problem.

The three most important compounds used up until 1988 were papaverine, phentolamine (Regitine), and phenoxybenzamine, since followed by prostaglandin E-1, VIP (vasoactive intestinal polypeptide), and thymoxamine (Virag, 1982; Zorgniotti & Lefleur, 1985; Brindley, 1983; Ishii et al., 1986; Ottesen et al., 1984; Buvat et al., 1989).

PAPAVERINE

Papaverine hydrochloride is considered the classic example of a prototype of nonspecific antispasmodic (relaxant) compounds. It is an alkaloid that occurs in about one percent of crude opium, but is chemically unrelated to the narcotic alkaloids and contributes nothing to the pharmacological effects of opium.

Under laboratory conditions, papaverine can relax all smooth muscles containing structures, irrespective of how the contraction has been induced.

It has been marketed for more than half of this century as tablets or in solutions for intramuscular or intravenous use in conditions of spasms (or colics) in gastrointestinal or urinary tracts, as well as for menstrual cramps or labor pains. More recently the compound has been used during surgery to relax and dilate arteries, as well as by radiologists when performing arteriography.

At the cellular level, through enzyme inhibition it is able to increase the level of cAMP (cyclic adenosinmonophosphate), which decreases the intracellular level of calcium. However, several other calcium regulations are affected, such as blocking the influx through the calcium channels of the cell membrane, inhibiting the intracellular release from calcium stores, and increasing the efflux of calcium from the smooth muscle cell.

Since calcium is the key in contraction and relaxation of the cells, its regulation is crucial to the function and the actual state of the smooth muscle cell, contracted or relaxed. As papaverine acts at several levels at the same time, it knocks out the smooth muscle completely, although in a reversible manner.

It affects all penile structures containing smooth muscle elements: the arteries, the cavernosal trabecular tissue, and the veins. Actually, through these actions it also reinforces the fact that the maintenance of rigidity is due to the so-called veno-occlusive mechanism, which all occurs inside the cavernous bodies (Andersson et al., 1991).

Papaverine may produce acute or chronic side effects, locally or systemically.

A. *Priapism, or prolonged erection, may persist even after one or several ejaculations.* It presents as a persistent hard erection that is unaffected by any external stimuli that normally will elicit penile detumescence.

It is unpredictable at which dose this may occur in a given patient and, therefore, requires close attention by the physician who injects intracavernosally. See below for further discussion.

B. Systemically papaverine may cause acute cardiovascular reactions such as slight cardiac irregularity and hypotension. Such reactions will usually not occur with doses used for intracavernous injections.

C. Local chronic damage may occur. This will be observed mostly as "nodules" in the cavernous tissue. This may be seen after a single injection, but usually after some months of use of the drug. The reason for this is not known.

However, the pH of the papaverine in solution is as low as 3, which is much lower than the normal 7.3 of the blood. If a blood sample is mixed with a few drops of a papaverine solution, a milky solution occurs as a result of precipitation of the drug because of the buffering ability of the blood.

Whether this precipate, which might occur after intracavernous injection, could be the cause of the nodules is not known. In rare instances, the nodules may persist and be felt as plaques as in Peyronie's Disease.

The reason for this is not known since such patients might naturally have developed the plaques anyhow during the treatment as a result of an ongoing development from an early, not detectable stage of the disease. Only extensive and refined diagnostic imaging techniques may in the future solve such questions as to the degree and extent of an early stage of fibrosis.

D. Any compound foreign to the body has to be eliminated. When papaverine is injected into the vascular system, it has a half-life of 1–2 hours in the blood. It is mainly metabolized in the liver and may cause a detectable increase in liver transaminases (which also can be seen after intake of alcohol).

More serious, but very uncommon, is a drug-induced hepatitis.

Patients who do not obtain full erection after injection of papaverine into the cavernous body will appear to have a higher systemic blood concentration, most likely due to failure of the cavernous closure system.

Due to these side effects of papaverine and the evidence of the efficacy of other drugs, the use of papaverine for self-injections seems to be on a decline (Jünemann et al., 1991).

ALPHA-ADRENOCEPTOR BLOCKADE

As noted earlier, a constant activity in the adrenergic nerves leads to a steady contraction (tonus) of the smooth muscles of the cavernous bodies due to release of norephinephrine, which contracts the smooth muscle cell and thereby keeps the penis flaccid.

Noradrenaline occurs to a great extent in the cavernous tissue. If sympathomitic drugs are applied, such as ephedrine, to prevent nasal congestion, an increase in the tone occurs and thereby lessened ability to relax the smooth muscles, making it difficult for the patient to obtain an erection. In contrast, systemic administrations of alpha-adrenoceptor blocking agents may lead to erection (like that reported with prazosin) or even to priapism. For this reason, the British physiologist Brindley tested local applications into the cavernous tissue, first applying phentolamine and later phenoxybenzamine.

Phenoxybenzamine

Phenoxybenzamine is a compound widely applied in the middle of this century as it was one of the first potent alpha-adrenoceptor antagonists that had a slow onset and a prolonged action, making it an acceptable compound for oral intake in the treatment of arterial hypertension. It has an effect on alpha-1, as well as on alpha-2 receptors, but in such a way that it binds itself irreversibly to the receptors on the cell surface by conjugation. This makes the compound questionable for clinical application when it is used locally in a high concentration, as it prevents, for a (long) period of time, restoration of normal responsiveness of the cells to the natural component norephedrine to induce detumescence.

New receptors have to be synthesized, which, together with the extremely long half-life of phenoxybenzamine, explains its very effective but unattractively long duration of relaxation of the smooth muscles of the cavernous tissue. The use of the compound gave rise to several cases of prolonged erection. Furthermore, systemic effects such as postural hypotension, tachycardia, and cardiac arrhythmias, as well hyperventilation, nausea, and cerebrally induced motoric excitability, make phenoxybenzamine unacceptable for the purpose of inducing erection.

In addition, it has been shown to be carcinogenic in animal experiments. Therefore, phenoxybenzamine has been discarded as a drug of choice, however powerful it might be in producing an erection.

Phentolamine

Phentolamine is another alpha-adrenoceptor antagonist that exerts an equal effect upon alpha-1 and alpha-2 adrenoceptors. However, it also blocks serotonin receptors. It has a direct relaxant effect upon the cells, as well. Its effect is reversible. The drug has a short plasma-halflife (30 min.), although there is a local effect of up to four hours duration. It is metabolized before excretion, but is not known to be hepatotoxic. Orally, it is ineffective in inducing penile erection as it is extensively metabolized after intestinal absorption.

Phentolamine's major effect upon the penile structures after intracavernous injection seems to be a decrease of the arterial inflow resistance (dilatation of arteries), with a much lesser effect on the outflow regulation. Usually, injection with phentolamine alone will not produce a full erection when this is the only stimulus. However, in combination with papaverine, prostaglandin E-1, or VIP, it is highly effective.

Thymoxamine

Thymoxamine is a relatively selective alpha-1 adrenoceptor blocking agent. It is less effective *in vitro* in reducing the tension of the norephinephrine precontracted tissue than phentolamine and papaverine on a weight-to-weight basis.

In animal experiments (dogs), it has shown an effect quite similar to phentolamine in reducing the arterial resistance, but has not been particularly effective in reducing the outflow. On this basis one might speculate whether we have sufficient knowledge about "selectivity" of alpha-receptors and if the hitherto accepted type-classification of the receptors is detailed enough. Subtypes classified as A, B and C among the alpha-1-receptors have recently been described in various tissues around the body.

Most recently, experimental work has shown type A as well as type B to exist in cavernous smooth muscles. This is indicative of a possible much more specific and rational approach to selecting the correct agent for a given pathophysiological situation in the future.

Some newly developed but not yet marketed highly specific and selective alpha-1-blocking agents seem to be effective and clinically useful in restoring erectile function when needed.

Prostaglandin E_1 (PGE$_1$).

PGE$_1$ is naturally occurring in many tissues of the body, including the cavernous tissue. It is synthesized with the generic name alprostadil and marketed as Prostin VR® (Upjohn, globally) and Prostavasin® (Schwarz-Pharma, Germany). It is registered for use in keeping the ductus arteriosus open in congenital heart disorders in newborns and for dilating in peripheral vascular (arterial) disease. Systemically, it produces vasodilatation, stimulates intestinal activity, and prevents platelet aggregation.

PGE$_1$ relaxes *in vitro* penile smooth muscle that has been precontracted by either prostaglandin $F_2\alpha$ or norepinephrine. When injected intracorporally in the penis, it produces erection.

Systemic side-effects almost never occur when it is injected intracavernosally as up to 90 percent of PGE$_1$ is metabolized in the lungs at one passage. Locally, it does not give rise to any known changes when used chronically and long-duration erections of more than four hours are very rare.

However, a number of men get pain when PGE_1 is injected and the pain will usually stay for the whole duration of erection. These men are not suitable for self-injection using PGE_1. The cause of the pain is not known, but it has been speculated that the injected PGE_1 interferes with the pain-sensitive nerves since the prostaglandins are involved in a still not understood way in metabolism of sensory nerves.

Other vasoactive compounds, some of which are naturally occurring but not registered for clinical use, have been tried. One is vasoactive intestinal polypeptide (VIP), which is very active *in vitro*. Injected intracavernosally in normal, potent men, it results in tumescence and, in a few men a short-lasting erection. In men who are impotent due to arterial insufficiency, doses as high as 60 micgr. do not elicit erection until further stimulation (vibration or visual sexual stimulation) is added. Doses in that range may cause nausea and pronounced flushing of the skin (Wagner & Gerstenberg, 1987). However, if the dose is decreased and phentolamine added, it seems to be clinically useful (Gerstenberg et al., 1991).

Calcitonin gene-related peptide (CGRP) is another potent vasodilatator. Although not very effective *in vitro* with muscle strips, it gives rise to a dose-related increase in arterial inflow and initiates the veno-occlusive mechanism resulting in erection (Stief et al., 1990).

Other compounds have been studied for their possible effect upon erection, such as calcium-channel blockers and potassium channel openers. Both types of drugs are effective *in vitro*, but systemic side effects seem to be an inhibiting factor for their clinical use (Giraldi & Wagner, 1990; Andersson et al., 1991).

Interactions between any of the used or suggested drugs used for penile erection have not been reported until very recently. In a case report of a 47-year-old man with multiple sclerosis, confined to a wheelchair, it was found that when he took amantidine, known as an antiviral or an antiparkinsonian agent, his intracorporal injections of prostaglandin-E_1 were completely ineffective. Without amantidine intake, prostaglandin-E_1 was highly effective (Earle et al., 1991).

CHAPTER IV

Diagnosis

by Gorm Wagner

ALTHOUGH MORE THAN 15 years have elapsed since a series of new investigative methods has been developed, the lack of standardization and of full knowledge as to the meaning of a "pathologic" finding still poses a problem.

Up until the late 1970s, it was considered "a truth" that 90 percent of patients complaining of erectile dysfunction had a psychogenic etiology. The rest of the patients were considered as suffering from organic causes arising from traumas, severe endocrine conditions, chronic illness and/or heavy medication.

With the realization that ordinary clinical assessment did not necessarily reveal any local organic components, it became clear that specific investigations would be necessary to come closer to a more differentiated understanding of the problem.

In our technical world, however, it has often been forgotten that a proper "old-fashioned" medical history is essential, and the area of erectile dysfunction is no exception. Basically, otherwise medically qualified persons are often not competent and knowledgable enough to take a professional history on another person's sexual function. Very few medical schools in the U.S. and Europe offer formalized training in sexology and unfortunately there has been a decline in the existing training during the last decade in spite of the acknowledged necessity of attending to *sexual health*, as declared by the World Health Organization in 1974.

As our sexuality is so closely woven into our personal cultural background, it is necessary to arrive at a more broad-minded and desensitized view of sexuality. It is this objective view that ideally forms the base for technical medical knowledge which, together with a widened understanding of sexuality, creates the professional medical interviewer.

An orthopedic surgeon who sees a patient with pain in the hip takes a quite detailed technical history of, for instance, in which positions, time of day, working situations, etc., etc., the pain occurs.

However, when it comes to complaints concerning the functioning of the sex organs in situations where they are supposed to function only under very private conditions of emotion, love, or pleasure, the detailed inquiry to elucidate this situation may easily come to an awkward halt, especially when differences in cultural and social backgrounds between the professional and the patient are evident. In addition, simple lack of courage as to "how far can I actually go in my questioning without offending my patient" may impede a professional attitude and in the end reduce the quality of a professional conclusion.

The point is that it is essential to have an open discussion of every detail as to how the patient's penis functions in all situations. History-taking is not quantifiable, except possibly for questionnaires. The value of taking a proper medical history when a patient is consulting for the first time actually cannot be quantified. We have to believe in the statements put forward by experienced physicians that a thorough medical history is the principal means to understand and evaluate the patient's situation before any decisions are made. Through the history alone, an experienced physician with sexological education will be able to establish a fairly correct diagnosis. For a more detailed discussion of sexual history, the reader is referred to Chapter VI.

To obtain diagnostic leads or to exclude not easily detectable conditions, technical tests such as blood samples, X-ray, ultrasound, and sophisticated neurological examinations may support or eliminate a diagnostic track previously set at the first verbal consultation. However, test results should be viewed with caution as we use them to formulate better questions and through an intellectual process draw more accurate conclusions.

As the diagnostic procedures have developed over a little more than a decade, we have seen seemingly good methods proposed, discussed, and then discarded. Often, a suggested method that seems to be useful in one clinic is found to be of less interest by other investigators.

Therefore, at the present time it is not possible to find a common denominator as to which single test is best out of the many possible tests suggested at meetings and in the medical literature. As a result of this lack of uniformity, it is impossible to set a fixed schedule for a "correct" algorithm of tests as no such agreement exists among the clinics and university centers around the world.

CURRENT DIAGNOSTIC TESTS

Impotence (erectile dysfunction) is not a clinical entity, but rather a symptom. At one time, a dysfunctional heart was described as morbus cordis (disease of the heart), a description that is unacceptable today in its lack of precision. But a dysfunctional penis is still accepted as a diagnosis since we have not yet managed to classify the etiologies and pathologies precisely enough to initiate a proper diagnostic classification and the use of proper nomenclature.

Basically, the very simplistic view that the cause of erection difficulties must be either psychologic or organic is nonsense. Several investigators have been able to identify at least two causative factors in a large proportion of patients. Often, two organic causes are demonstrable and frequently a psychological component will be added to this even though it is not always possible to detect at which point it appeared, to what degree it has interfered, and whether or not it is an *effect* of the erectile failure or a *cause* of it.

Recently, the French internist Jacques Buvat stated: "there continue to be two irreconcilable groups of therapists dealing with erectile dysfunction, the 'organic' group, including physicians and particularly surgeons, who think of erectile function only in hydraulic terms, who take even the most minor physical abnormality in a diagnostic test as evidence of 'organic' causation, and who assume that in most other cases this is a concealed physical cause waiting to be identified. Their clinical approach is preoccupied with establishing indications for surgical treatment. The 'psychogenic' group, on the other hand, see symbolic somatic manifestations of psychic conflicts in every organic disease and deny any primary organic aetiology in erectile dysfunction. The literature remains cluttered with studies from the organic group based on questionable methodology, lacking appropriate controls, leading to subjective conclusions, whilst the psychogenic group continue with their anecdotal reports of single cases or at best very small uncontrolled studies" (Buvat et al., 1990).

After the medical history is completed, the patient is asked to lie down supine on the examination table. The first important and simple procedure is to conduct a thorough palpation of the penis, as described on p. 43, Chapter II. This can be followed by one or more of the tests described below.

Doppler Investigation

An 8 MH_3 Doppler probe with or without stethoscope can be used with auscultation to identify the femoral vessels. The dorsal arteries should be identified as well. With the glans pointed towards the abdomen, the deep arteries can be identified at the base of the penis. Due to substantial differences in anatomy, it may not be possible in normal men to locate, for instance, only one of the four penile arteries. But what is more important to realize is that in some patients, as well as in young volunteers with normal erection, Doppler auscultation of all four arteries is not always possible. The type of patient in whom most often auscultation is not possible may commonly end up classified as "psychogenic." In a young/younger man with a firm and extremely contracted cavernous body, the arteries will also be maximally contracted, most probably due to a high adrenergic activity.

Unfortunately, we do not have any diagnostic procedure to evaluate the acute systemic level of the activity in the sympathetic system. It may very well be that some persons have a tendency for a high sympathetic tone in certain organ systems. This would not be occurring in other parts of the sympathetic system and, therefore, would not be detectable as a generalized reaction. A negative (non audible) response to a Doppler examination is of value if a similar test is conducted shortly after an intracavernous injection of a vasoactive substance and the arteries then become audible with a normal sound of dilation. A positive response to Doppler examination of the flaccid penis tells us that the arteries are not obstructed.

If a wave-form analysis is coupled to the Doppler system, it is possible to obtain a chart-strip recording. However, it has clearly been shown that the wave form is closely related to the angle at which the probe is held to the axis of flow in the artery and how far from an existing stenosis the probe is positioned. On this basis, reproducibility by use of this technique is low, as is the sensitivity (Meuleman et al., 1990).

High-resolution ultrasonography combined with pulsed Doppler spectrum analysis (duplex scanning), which is possible only in special institutions due to the high cost of the equipment, makes it possible to measure the blood flow velocities in the individual arteries and the diameter of the vessels, as well as to scan the corpora for fibrotic lesions. The reliability of the method in the flaccid state is low (Lue et al., 1985, 1986).

After intracavernous injection (ICI) has been given, a pronounced dilatation and an increase in blood velocity will be seen within a period of three to five minutes. A systolic peak-velocity of more than 25 cm/min and an increase of more than 75 percent of diameter is indicative of no arterial insufficiency of the cavernous arteries. If erection occurs at this stage, vascular disease is not probable. If no erection occurs in spite of a well-established reaction of the arterial system, it is likely that a veno-occlusive dysfunction is causing the erectile problem.

Only recently, these methods have been tried experimentally in men without erectile dysfunction and the results indicate that even lower values as mentioned above (as lower normal values) can be found in normals. As the psychological state of the patient during the investigation may influence the response to ICI, it can be expected that the method may render false positive results (Schwartz et al., 1989).

Penile Blood Pressure (PBP)

The arterial blood pressure of the penis is measured by applying a small (finger) cuff around the base of the penis. Most simple is to use an ordinary blood pressure apparatus equipped with a bulb or, even easier to handle, a syringe by which a more stable pressure can be kept when listening for the systolic pressure sound. A simple Doppler on one of the audible arteries can be used for the sound detection. No studies of the pressures of the four individual arteries seem to exist. Therefore, ideally one of the deep penile arteries should be selected as most representative, as these arteries are mainly responsible for the erectile functions.

An automatic apparatus that is self-inflating and deflating and measures the systolic and diastolic pressure as well as calculating the mean pressure, using the oscillation principle, is convenient since other examinations can be performed simultaneously. The pressure obtained and averaged after three measurements is compared with similar measurement of the pressure of the index finger.

A penile "brachial" blood pressure index, PBPI, is calculated based on either the systolic or the mean pressure, which do not differ significantly.

An index of 0.1–0.6 is indicative of arterial insufficiency. Sometimes, no pressure can be obtained, which frequently will be caused by a situational closure of the arteries to such an extent that the cuff, strain gauge, or Doppler cannot detect even the systolic pressure. An index above 0.8 is considered as being yielded by normal arteries.

The method has a high specificity, but low sensitivity, and may therefore give false positives, but rarely false negatives (Alter et al., 1988; Buvat et al., 1988).

Another simple method is to use a mercury strain-gauge—as used in ordinary testing on a finger or toe—to study the wave-form where a fast upstroke and existence of a dicrotic notch are indicative of normal arteries (Zorgniotti & Lizza, 1991).

Three to five minutes after injection of a standard dose of a vasoactive compound, the Doppler sound will increase, usually along with the blood pressure and the plethysmographic curve, all indicative of responding arteries.

If all these tests of the arteries are indicative of arteriogenic insufficiency and the medical history points in this direction, the time has come to consider whether or not further invasive studies should be carried out. This can be decided only after a thorough discussion with the patient to find out whether he, if a phalloarteriography gives indication for it, is willing to undergo vascular surgery with the intention of revascularizing the corpora cavernosa. Other possibilities, such as the use of a vacuum device, surgically implanted penile prosthesis, or trial with increasing doses of erection-producing injections should be discussed at this point. The patient should be urged not to make a hasty decision but rather to take time to think it over and, if possible, discuss this in depth with his spouse as well. He should be encouraged to return for further discussion on unresolved questions.

Sometimes a man may choose to stop further investigations at this stage. He may feel satisfied after a thorough examination and even relieved that a probable cause for his problem has been found.

Biochemical Screening

Glucose in urine, blood lipids/cholesterol, and serum prolactin seem to be the most common routine examinations of body fluids. It may be that an undetected case of diabetes mellitus will be disclosed and normal procedures to correct the biochemical status may in some cases lead to normalization of the erectile disorder without further interference.

On rare occasions a (very) high prolactin is found; if so, specialized endocrinological treatment should be sought. Once the prolactin is normalized some patients may regain their ability to erect (Buvat et al., 1990). It is not understood why a high prolactin level may influence erectile function.

Diet-changes due to high serum lipids/cholesterol or stopping smoking in heavy smokers will contribute more to good general health than it will to improving the erectile ability within any short period of time. However, some few cases who are hypersensitive to nicotine will regain potency less than one week after the last cigarette (Forsberg et al., 1979).

Pharmaco-Cavernosometry

An artificial erection created by infusion of normal saline into the cavernous bodies by an infusion pump, hand-held syringe, or gravity, after ICI of papaverine has been administered and where the flow to maintain a constant pressure is measured, is called pharmacocavernosometry.

If a large flow, i.e. more than 30 ml/min is necessary to maintain the pressure of erection, it is indicative of a leaking system. This can be caused by a general insufficient veno-occlusive mechanism or by one or several large veins that drain directly from the cavernous body.

False positives may occur up to a value of 100 ml/min, as it has been shown that normal men, as well as proven psychogenic cases, may come out with high values as well (Buvat et al., 1989b; Fuchs et al., 1989). If a high maintenance flow rate is found and the procedure is done on an X-ray table contrast medium can be injected into the cavernous body to visualize from where the high outflow occurs.

At the meeting in Rio in 1990 of the International Society of Impotence Research, several surgeons reported on the outcome of venous surgery, including many new technical modifications. More than 2500 surgically treated patients were reported on. The overall conclusion was that whichever technique is used the basic problem is to identify the right diagnostic work-up. This should be based on which pathological cause is creating the problem of too much leaking from the high pressure area of the cavernous bodies during erection (Int. J. Impotence Res. Suppl. 2, 1990).

Visual Sexual Stimulation

Other methods for early diagnostic work-up have been suggested. In *Visual Sexual Stimulation* (VSS), one or more sequences of erotic scenes are shown to the patient, who is seated in a room by himself in front of a TV monitor. His penile response is recorded either through a strain-gauge or by a TV camera. If he develops a full erection through this stimulation, no further tests are needed (Wagner & Green, 1981).

The method is of value only if positive since it may be negative even in young, normal men. Older men with no erectile problems are less likely to respond than younger men. The method is not feasible in all cultures, but quite often the resistance to using this simple method may come from the institution or the diagnostician rather than from the patient. In some states it may even be illegal.

Vibration

This is another simple method whereby a full erection can be induced in normal young men, in psychogenic patients, and in spinal-cord injured if the lesion is at the thoracic level or higher. If no erection occurs, the test has no value.

The man is placed seated with his penis lying on the vibrating device. He regulates the amplitude and frequency himself on a control panel. He is told not to exceed a frequency of 70 h_3 as this frequency and higher easily may result in ejaculation. Three minutes of self-regulated vibration are sufficient to determine the effect. If full erection occurs, no vascular insufficiency exists, nor does any local neurological disorder, sensory or motor (Wagner, 1985).

Vibration combined with VSS is more effective than each of the two stimuli alone (Wagner & Gerstenberg, 1987). Again, if a fully developed erection results under this condition, no further test procedures are necessary.

Nocturnal Penile Tumescence (NPT)

When NPT is combined with monitoring of rigidity (NPTR), the penile erections, which are associated with the REM-sleep phases, can be quantified. The value of the test is still under debate, especially as some investigators have found "abnormal" NPTR in normal young persons and because the tests in a sleep lab are expensive and may have to be repeated for several nights if the first night is "abnormal" (Kirkeby et al., 1989; Buvat et al., 1990). Portable instruments for home use do exist and reduce the cost of the test.

The majority of older men have "abnormal" NPT even if they are normally functioning. Thus, the standardization of this method is insufficient. Only a fully "normal" recording can be accepted as indicative of a non-organic cause. However, normal NPTR may be seen in dysfunctionally erectile patients with spinal cord injury or with pelvic-steal-syndrome patients, who experience completely normal rigid erection when stimulated sexually, but lose the erection as soon as coital movements with pelvic thrusting begin.

Equally important is the fact that so far no one has been able to identify which part(s) of the autonomic nerve systems are involved in the existence of nocturnal tumescence periods. Could it be due to a combination of inhibition of spontaneous, myogenic activity and a local complete block of adrenergic nervous tone, a situation that might not be absolutely similar to the occurrence of normal erection? Thus far, nobody has been able to explain why urination at the peak of the morning rigidity makes the penis flaccid almost immediately.

It is well established that the morning erection as such is unrelated to the degree of filling of the bladder (Wagner & Green, 1981).

Again, crucial basic questions on how to explain a normal physiological phenomenon like NPT are still able to shatter the clinical interpretation.

Hence, no single test to pinpoint the etiology of the symptom of erectile dysfunction is acceptable. Once more, we may conclude that the art of combining clinical observation with simple non-invasive or semi-invasive procedures may give a fairly good basis for a diagnostic decision that will be followed by a suggestion for a treatment.

More research is clearly needed.

CHAPTER V

Injection Therapy for Impotence

by Gorm Wagner

GUIDE TO USE OF INJECTIONS

When should the Intracavernosal Pharmaco-Injection Be Used?

The initial concept was to use papaverine as office injections at intervals to improve the natural erections, serving much like a repetitive "cure." (Virag, 1982). At present, the vasoactive compounds are used in the following five situations:

1. During the early phase of medical evaluation, as a diagnostic test;
2. During cavernosometry in searching for a leakage from the cavernous body, and later during the radiological examination, cavernosography;
3. For evaluation of men who, with or without a concomitant Peyronie's Disease, develop a curvature during erection and who are not able to produce a photo for the surgeon to decide which strategy to use for the surgical correction of the bending(s);

4. For occasional patients who, after a single diagnostic test-injection, significantly improve for a period. Such patients may benefit from occasional office injections, often with 2-3 month intervals;
5. For self-injection after medical diagnostic evaluation and instruction. This is to be used before intercourse takes place.

Which Drug and What Dose?

As this development is so recent and as it is based on a steadily growing body of clinical experience in regard to safety and efficacy, it would be unwise to recommend any of the possibilities shown in Table V.1 as being the best. A physician would be best advised to start with a single compound and then gradually work towards the composed solution. The experienced physician will know that it is difficult to stick to a fixed procedure in any individual clinical situation.

TABLE V.1
Marketed Drugs That Have Been/Are
Used for ICI, Although Registered
for Other Indications.

1982	papaverine
1983	phenoxybenzamine
1984	papaverine/phentolamine
1986	prostaglandin E_1 (PGE_1)
1989	thymoxamine
1990	PGE_1/phentolamine
1991	papaverine/PGE_1/phentolamine

Who May Benefit?

If a patient, after thorough explanation of different options, makes the decision to try self-injection, this should be done on the basis of the highest possible level of technical and pedagogic information to avoid practical, medical, and psychological problems and to make it less likely that the patient will drop the treatment due to lack of information.

For further discussion on compliance and the "therapeutic alliance" between doctor and patient, see Chapter IV. Following are types of cases who may benefit from intracavernous injections (ICI):

Mild cases of arteriogenic etiology;
All cases of neurogenic etiology;
Selected cases of psychogenic etiology;
Mild cases of abnormal leakage;
Unresolved cases, and in cases who have had unsuccessful (or partly successful) venous surgery.

Severe cases of abnormal leakage and severe cases of mixed vascular are the two groups who usually will not respond to any of the drug combinations. Such patients should rather be considered candidates for surgery: venous ligation (Lue, 1988), arterial revascularization (DePalma et al., 1988; Levine & Goldstein, 1990), or penile implant (Gerstenberg, et al., 1979; Krane, 1988; Pedersen et al., 1988).

If surgery is contraindicated or not wanted by the patient, he can be taught the use of a vacuum device, as this method is simple and safe if used properly (Nadig, 1989). The principle consists of reducing the atmospheric pressure around the penis when it is placed in an airtight chamber. This makes the blood fill all vessels and cavernous spaces and the penis will grow into a size of normal erection or sometimes a little larger. Then, a rubber band is rolled around the base of the penis and the airtight cylinder removed. It is a method that has been used in India and the Far East from ancient times, as an intermittent treatment in certain clinics as prevention of losing potency.

SELECTING THE DRUG

Once the decision has been made to try the symptomatic treatment of the erectile dysfunction in order to induce an erection on demand, the objective is to find the smallest possible dose.

Different approaches have been suggested to solve this problem since the response to a given dose in the office may very well differ from the response to the same dose when the patient is with his partner. One method is to escalate the dose to a level that produces an erection in the office and then prescribe a 10-30 percent *lower* dose to be used at home. Most commonly, the situation in the private setting will be more stimulating than that in the office.

If a weaker compound is used, such as thymoxamine or phentolamine alone, these drugs will rarely by themselves produce a full erection in the office. Rather, they *facilitate* the development of an erection under normal home conditions purely as a pharmaceutical support. However, it has to be discussed with the patient if he is willing to try this approach even knowing that it may fail. The reason for being cautious with this approach is that if the patient is not prepared for one or two early failures, he, or the couple, may lose confidence in the self-injection method.

A third method is the use of stimulation in the office after injection. As discussed under the diagnostic procedures, visual sexual stimulation or vibration or the combination of the two has been suggested. The simplest of the two is vibration. After the injection the patient lies supine for 10 minutes, then is allowed to stand or sit for five minutes, followed by three minutes of vibration, which is regulated by the patient himself. In 90 percent of cases who have a good initial response to the intracavernous medication, a further increase in volume and development of rigidity will occur during the three-minute vibration period (Wagner, 1985). This gives the patient sufficient information as to the development of rigidity to the point where it is sufficient for vaginal penetration. It also assures him that his own body is participating in the process and that external stimuli should be part of the lovemaking.

The mechanical vibration is preferred to self-masturbation as the latter is less controllable and may even be resisted by the patient without his telling the physician. The advantage for the diagnostician is obvious because the individual case can be evaluated under standardized circumstances. To ask the patient to rush home to perform a coital trial cannot be recommended as a standard procedure.

Patients who have achieved a good erectile response during the first consultation may occasionally ask: "May I use it now after I leave your office?" No objection should be made to his doing so. Rather, the response might be: "You are welcome, but you don't have to" and the decision left to the patient.

When a patient has had a first office-injection and if he

on this occasion develops a full rigid erection, some clinics require that he remain until the erection has shown signs of subsiding. No universal rules can be given as how to handle this best. It must depend on the patient/doctor relationship, on distances, on time of day, etc. Ideally, a fixed time (for instance, four hours later) is decided for telephone contact between the doctor and the patient for a brief communication on the state of the penis.

This is recommended in all situations even if the patient leaves the office with no rigidity.

The reason for this is that most cases of prolonged erection occur after the first diagnostic injection regardless of which compound or combinations are used. Five to 10 percent of prolonged erections were reported in the first studies, which then resulted in doctors reducing the initial dose and increasing the titrating doses more slowly. However, this makes several more visits to the clinic/office necessary and may on this ground put some patients off (Jünemann & Alken, 1989).

The incidence of prolonged erection after the first visit has now dropped to a few percent and lower. However, it still occurs in some patients, particularly in those who may have a neurogenic cause. The reason for this is not fully understood, nor can a neurogenic case always be detected on the first visit (Jünemann & Alken, 1989).

In addition to having direct access to the injecting physician during the first hours after the injection, the patient should either have access to a 24-hour telephone service or be instructed as to which emergency clinic he could turn to in event of persistent erection. Not all emergency rooms are well prepared for reducing a penile erection.

Several methods have been suggested to treat a pharmacologically induced persistent erection (priapism) (Jünemann & Alken, 1989).

In one method, a puncture of the cavernous body is made with a 21 gauge needle and blood is withdrawn into a syringe 20–80 ml. As a result, the erection sometimes disappears, and then may resume. Saline with a vasoconstrictor is then introduced and can be withdrawn using a flushing technique.

However, as a first attempt it is most simple to inject either phenylephrine or epinephrine (only 20 micrograms) in 0.1 ml at the base and the top of the shaft and then wait. This can be repeated after 20–30 minutes. It takes longer to be effective, but is not as bloody as the withdrawal method. These two agents are safe in the doses recommended above. Previously metaraminol was recommended but it is a drug with longer action and runs the risk of overdose. Cases have been reported with hypertensive crisis after the use of metaraminol in treatment of prolonged erection.

The preferred agent used today is prostaglandin E_1 (PGE_1), most often as a one ml injection of a 10 microgram per ml solution. Studies comparing papaverine versus papaverine/phentolamine versus PGE_1 have shown the superiority of PGE_1 as most effective. The main problem in using PGE_1 is, however, that 10 to 20 percent of the patients get pain in the cavernous bodies. The pain persists until the erection has completely subsided (Jünemann & Alken, 1989).

The pain may be mild or severe and one cannot predict which patient will experience it. There seems to be a tendency to less pain if the concentration is lowered, i.e. To use a solution of 10 micrograms per two ml. Usually, the cases of weak pain may respond to an aspirin. Some clinical reports indicate that those who have weak pain (not preventing intercourse) may experience a gradual disappearance of the pain after a few self-injections. However, a good doctor/patient relationship is necessary to convince a patient to try this road without losing confidence in the method. In some patients, the drug is so painful that it prevents erection. Unfortunately, it cannot be tested for beforehand. Therefore, the patient must be informed about this possibility before injecting.

This is very different from the burning sensation that some men feel after injection of papaverine. In these cases, the discomfort rarely is severe and is always brief, lasting, 60–120 seconds.

Those who experience pain after PGE_1 will not continue the self-injection program with this drug.

A simple way to continue is to prepare a solution of 4 microgram of PGE_1 and 1 milligram of phentolamine (Regitine) per ml and using one ml of this solution. Clinical experience reported at scientific meetings but not in any published studies tells us that there have been no cases of painful reaction using this combination.

More and more patients who have been using papaverine or papaverine/phentolamine are now shifted to PGE_1 or its combination with phentolamine. This changeover arises either from the patient's own request or from the physician's initiative as PGE_1 injections over longer periods have been found to give fewer fibrotic reactions. This also reduces the number of control-visits for palpation check up.

One disadvantage of the PGE_1 solution is that if kept in the refrigerator it has a full activity period of only three months and then gradually loses its activity. If kept at room temperature, the activity period is shorter. It is important to emphasize this to the patient.

INJECTION-TECHNIQUE

An area on the right or left side of the shaft stretching from 1 cm behind the glans to 1 cm from the base of the penis can be used. Depending on the diameter (size) of the flaccid penis, the width of these areas may vary from 5 to 10 millimeters. This gives sufficient space to select a spot with no visible vessels in or immediately under the skin. Therefore, a good light is necessary so as not to penetrate vessels. However, one cannot always avoid puncturing vessels deeper in the fat-free subcutaneous tissue among the fascias. For this reason, it is recommended that one presses a sponge to the area of puncture for one minute *after* needle withdrawal so as to prevent bleeding.

Figure V.1 shows the direction in which the needle should be inserted to avoid damage to nerves, vessels and urethra. When you are teaching the patient how to inject, he can be standing or sitting/reclining. Using sketches or instructional video facilitates the patient's understanding of where to inject (Figure V.2).

After the skin has been wiped properly with a sterilizing swab, the needle should be inserted in one short, firm movement at a 90-degree angle until it is in up to the hub. There are several types of disposable syringes on the market, but a disposable 1-ml syringe equipped with a 26-gauge (0.45 mm) ⅜ inch (10 mm) needle is ideal. This needle is large and strong enough to be withdrawn from a rubber-capped vial and small enough to be almost painless. The length is correct for this use as seen in Figure V.1.

Once the needle is inserted, the plunger can be pushed and no resistance should be felt. If resistance does occur, the needle should be withdrawn 1-(2) mm and injection can be tried again. If there is still resistance, the needle

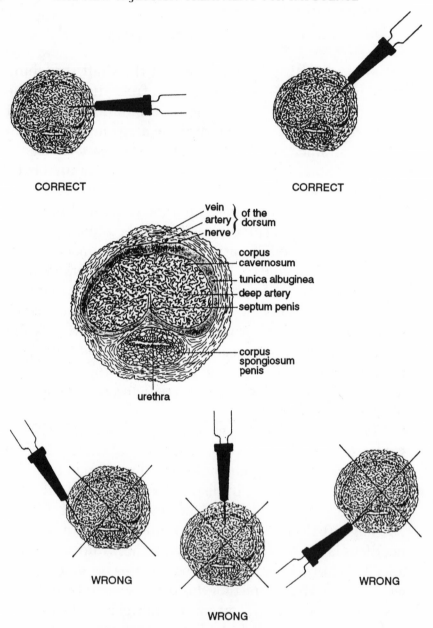

Figure V.1   Cross-section of the shaft of the penis to demonstrate the correct angle of the needle and where not to inject. Scale 1:1.

should be completely removed and a droplet should be pushed through to check for obstruction. After this, another attempt at insertion can be made.

It is simplest for the patient to try the whole technical procedure of withdrawing from the vial (or the ampoule), doing the proper cleaning, learning how to handle the syringe and needle, removing air from the barrel, etc. with the instructor sitting next to him. Then he can insert the needle into an object like a citrus fruit or an onion, which gives some feel of how easy it is to carry out the injection and what type of resistance is met.

Some physicians massage the shaft for a short period after injections in order to facilitate contact between the tissue and the compound. The use of a tourniquet around the base of the penis during and for three minutes after the injection has been suggested. This may prevent the drug from escaping too fast, especially if there is a high outflow, and in this way prevent any untoward systemic effects from the injected compound (Wagner, 1985).

Once the patient has been instructed in the whole procedure, he should demonstrate it all, including a self-injection using saline. It should also be explained that the injection may not be successful the first and second times and that it takes time to get accustomed to this procedure.

At some stage, the patient should be asked if he wants his partner to participate in the instruction and/or the discussion of how to live with this new situation. He should also be encouraged to consider further support such as counselling or supportive sex therapy. This is discussed elsewhere in this book.

There are probably as many ways to handle this new situation at home as there are individuals. At one extreme, the patient will hide it all from the partner and secretly

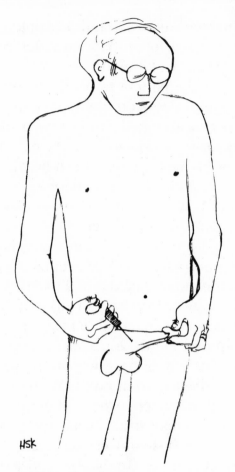

Figure V.2   Self-injection sketch.

inject himself before any initiation of lovemaking. At the other extreme, the spouse takes care of preparing the syringe and performs the injection whenever the occasion arises.

The duration of erection should ideally be only until an ejaculation/orgasm has occurred. If an effective dose of papaverine/phentolamine has been given and the lovemaking has had only a short duration, the erection will continue after ejaculation, but in a different way. Only the shaft will be rigid, whereas the glans and spongious body will lose their tumescence. Some patients describe this as an "odd" non-erotic feeling. If after some time they are able to be stimulated again and sexually (mentally) aroused, the tumescence of glans will return and it will be felt as a normal erection again.

With the use of PGE_1, this artificial situation seems to be eliminated as most patients experience a normal detumescence after ejaculation, although the actual volume (size) of the penis may be larger for a longer postcoital period than usual. Sometimes, it is possible to obtain another normal erection after some time, even for men who previously did not have this ability.

One cannot discuss with the patient all these possible details, which may or may not occur, before he has had some experience with the injection at home. One approach is to see the patient when he has used the self-injection technique five times, unless he has problems earlier. At this consultation, it can be discussed how the couple has reacted in the new situation and technical problems can be solved.

The patient should be advised not to inject himself more than twice a week, with a two day interval at least. This can be adjusted at the first control visit two to three months later when a penile physical examination should be carried out to ensure that no fibrotic changes have occurred.

As a clinical experience, it is occasionally noted that a return of erectile capability occurs after some months of self-injection treatment. Not until very recently has a study been conducted addressing this issue. The Australian urologist McMahon followed 153 men with erectile dysfunction who had started on a self-injection program using prostaglandin E_1. Ninety-four of these were diagnosed as mainly arteriogenic, 22 had cavernosal leakage, and 37 were psychogenic. A smaller, similarly composed group comprised an untreated control group. The patients were seen two, four, and six months after initiation of treatment.

Improved erections in the control group without injections were noted in 5–9 percent in the two groups of vascular cases and in 20 percent of the psychogenic cases. In the self-injection group, the study showed 6–13 percent improvement among the cases with vascular etiology. In the psychogenic group, however, 62 percent at four months and 85 percent at six months declared that their erections had improved and their potency had been restored.

This study suggests, therefore, that self-injection of prostaglandin E_1 is associated with restoration of potency only in patients with psychogenic and rarely in patients with organic impotence (McMahon, 1992).

There have been reports in the medical literature, up until 1992, of more than 4400 patients using papaverine, 4350 cases using papaverine and phentolamine, and more than 3000 cases using PGE_1.

The incidence of prolonged erection in self-injection programs is less than 0.5 percent based on more than 60,000 injections in 2356 patients using papaverine alone or in combination with phentolamine (0.3 percent) and over 9000 injections using PGE_1 in more than 1000 patients (0.2 percent).

In a study of the literature (Jünemann et al., 1991), a total of 482 cases were found who had been tested with several vasoactive agents. With papaverine, 35 percent of the men obtained full erection; papaverine/phentolamine was effective in 68 percent; and PGE_1 in 76 percent. Prolonged erections in this particular group of the retested men occurred in 3 percent using papaverine, 3.6 percent using papaverine/phentolamine, and in only 1 percent when PGE_1 was used in the same men.

CONTRAINDICATIONS

Any medical condition that involves *cardiac or vascular instability* (hypo- or hypertension) should be evaluated by a cardiologist before a self-injection program using any of the drugs is begun. As PGE_1 is the compound that has the least systemic effect, this is the drug of choice once the patient has been cleared by the cardiologist, who should be told what doses are to be used.

Other contraindications are:

Severe cirrhosis of the liver;
Severe abuse of drugs or alcohol;
Mental instability;
Conditions that may imply poor compliance;
Allergy to the compound or its solvents;
Tremor of hands or other physical disabilities, unless
    partner is trained;
Known sex-offenders.

SOME ETHICAL ISSUES

Some have raised the possibility of abuse of self-injection and suggested that any man who is to enter a self-injection program should be referred to a psychiatrist specializing in psychosexual medicine and have a proper assessment to ensure that "deviant," "disordered," or "dishonest" men are not allowed to enter such program (O'Gorman & Bownes, 1990).

If one should have to undergo such an assessment, it would be up to the evaluator to judge, based on his/her present moral/religious or societal conviction, who should be approved. It would be like refusing hand surgery to restore bending of the right index finger until a psychiatric evaluation could ensure that the finger would never pull a trigger.

I feel that any individual has the right to request injection therapy, regardless of his inner motives, and it is up to the individual physician to decide what is appropriate and serves his patient best. Any first meeting with a new patient has to deal with a number of sexual issues so as to reveal the patient's true motive for treatment.

Sometimes injection therapy is obviously inappropriate. For example, if the interview reveals the patient wants to get into an ICI program only to "refine" his erection or believes ICI may make his erection last for hours. Such a patient should be discouraged from having this treatment.

As with any other medical issue, the physician, after a thorough evaluation, must base the final decision both on his professional judgment and on the need of the patient.

A special problem was posed for American physicians in 1988 when a pharmaceutical company (Eli Lilly) labeled their papaverine vials: "Papaverine hydrochloride is not indicated for the treatment of impotence by intracavernous injection. The intracorporal injection of papaverine has been reported to have resulted in persistent priapism requiring medical and surgical intervention." This was, presumably, not done for moralistic reasons but rather to avoid possible lawsuits. However, the product is still man-ufactured and sold by the same company.

The injection technique has improved life quality for tens of thousands of couples around the world. This tech-nique has to be accepted until new approaches are devel-oped, either in the form of transdermal applications or by the oral route. As one patient who used papaverine told me: "My wife gets a certain glint in her eyes when she says at bedtime, 'let's go up and have some papa-virile!'"

CHAPTER VI

The Psychiatric Aspects of Injection Treatment

by Helen Singer Kaplan

INTRACAVERNOSAL INJECTION therapy is a major advance in sexual medicine that can enable many impotent men to attain erections that look and feel perfectly normal. However, some patients are unable to use or to derive long-term benefits from this marvelous new technology because of hidden emotional or marital difficulties.

Noncompliant patients attain satisfying erections when they receive an injection in the doctor's office. At this time, they often appear enthusiastic. However, after they take their premixed solution and their syringes home, they fail to take advantage of these to improve the frequency and the quality of their sexual relationships. Typically, the noncompliant patient will try the injections once or twice. But for reasons he cannot always articulate, he then leaves the material in the refrigerator and avoids sex altogether. Others are unable to translate their excellent pharmacologically induced erections into satisfying sexual experiences because their partners do not cooperate.

It can be puzzling and frustrating to the urologist when patients who seem so eager to regain their potency, and who are good responders in the doctor's office, resist and avoid using the injections to make love at home. But resistance is not unique to ICI programs. This is a ubiquitous phenomenon in the mental health field, and a great deal is known about the causes and management of resistance to psychotherapy. This expertise is applicable to minimizing the risks of noncompliance with pharmacotherapy and to helping patients overcome their resistances to this treatment.

REDUCING THE RISKS OF NONCOMPLIANCE

Psychiatrists and psychologists have been familiar with the concept of resistance to treatment since the turn of the century, when Freud described a seemingly paradoxical tendency for his patients in psychoanalysis to resist getting well (Freud, 1924). Freud's explanation of this phenomenon was that on some deeply unconscious level of the mind, certain people are threatened by success and sabotage themselves as a result of unresolved childhood problems. With some modifications, this theoretical formulation is still accepted today. Since that time, it has also become apparent that the phenomenon of resistance is not confined to psychoanalysis. In fact, this self-destructive form of behavior is so widespread that the management of resistance has become a central issue in many other forms of psychological treatment, including psychosexual therapy (Kaplan, 1979, 1987).

It has been fascinating to observe, in the course of combining sex therapy and injection therapy with noncompliant patients, that the same manifestations of resistance and the same sorts of dynamics that we see in psychogenically impotent patients who are in sex therapy can also arise in patients with medical erectile disorders who are undergoing pharmacological injection programs. Thus, both types of patients may sabotage the improvement of their sexual relationships, which is the goal of both treatments, by missing their appointments, botching up the doctor's instructions, antagonizing their partners, etc. For example, one of my patients left his paraphernalia in a taxi; another took a lengthy, "males only" fishing trip without his wife just when he was ready to begin using his injections with her.

The psychological issues that give rise to noncompliance in patients undergoing pharmacotherapy and those undergoing sex therapy are strikingly similar. In both types of treatment, the psychological causes of resistance range in severity from mild concerns that the patient recognizes to serious unconscious conflicts. More specifically, minor reasons for noncompliance include the simple (and normal) fear of injecting oneself into the penis, a mild concern that the partner will be put off by and object to his "artificial" erection, and some guilt about spending too much money and energy on one's sexual pleasure. On the other end of this continuum are severe intrapsychic and marital conflicts that result in the patient's ambivalence about sex. The latter are usually deeply rooted in painful childhood events.

Most of the patients referred to us because they experienced problems adapting to intracavernosal injection therapy were free of major psychopathology and their resistances fell into the minor category. However, even these mild or "superficial" sorts of resistances can result in complete treatment failures if they are not attended to properly.

In many cases, such minor psychological obstacles to compliance can be prevented or dispelled rapidly by the doctor's support and reassurance, along with a few positive experiences. But the physician should not give up if the patient continues to have difficulties despite his best efforts. Such situations can often be salvaged, even with more seriously disturbed patients, by collaboration with a therapist who is knowledgeable about sexual problems and skilled in managing resistance.

The following suggestions for preventing and minimizing noncompliance with ICI, grew out of our experience with patients who had problems using the injections.

The Therapeutic Alliance

A good working therapeutic relationship between the managing doctor* and the patient (or in some cases with both partners) can make the difference between a successful outcome and a treatment failure.

If the doctor acts in a supportive, encouraging manner that flows out of his understanding of and empathy with his patients' underlying feelings, patients are likely to develop positive transferences, which cause them to invest the doctor with almost magical omnipotence and omniscience. When they are in a positive transferential state,

---

*The "Managing Doctor" is not necessarily the physician who dispenses the injections, although, of course, he often is. However, if the man or his partner are especially difficult, or if the patient is already engaged in sex therapy, or if the urologist does not have the time, the personality, or the interest to develop a sound therapeutic alliance with his patients, a team approach often works best. The sex therapist or the patient's own psychiatrist is often in a better position to manage the case from a psychological viewpoint, while the injections and medical management are provided by the urologist.

patients become somewhat childlike. They put complete trust in their doctors, will suspend their own judgments, and make every effort to please him/her.

Such a strong positive transference can be extremely useful when the doctor is trying to persuade a frightened patient to jab a needle into his penis, to allay his anxiety about doing harm to his genitalia, to assuage his concerns about being humiliated in front of his partner, or to reassure a threatened wife that her husband is not going to use the injections to become promiscuous.

The symptoms of sexual inadequacy, as well as injections into the genitalia, are for most individuals highly emotional issues; patients undergoing this treatment tend to feel vulnerable. While extremely stable patients with loving, secure partners may need little psychological support and understanding, and will successfully adapt to the injections even if the physician maintains his distance, many men and their partners are not all that well integrated or motivated and they need the doctor's help to overcome their fears. For such fragile couples a strong therapeutic alliance is a crucial ingredient in the success of treatment.

When he has a positive transference, a patient is likely to turn to his doctor for help if he and his partner have problems adapting to the injections. This is quite common in the beginning even for patients who eventually make excellent adjustments. But if the doctor is in a hurry, or seems impatient with the patient's sometimes irrational anxieties, or seems annoyed by the patient's needs, which may seem excessive, for continual reassurance, or if he transmits his own discomfort with sex to the patient, the doctor/patient relationship is likely to be inadequate to the task.

If a patient does not feel safe with or understood by his doctor, he is not likely to call him should he experience difficulties. Patients who do not have faith in their doctors have nowhere to turn for support and they are apt to become discouraged and are likely to abandon the injections after a few problematic attempts. To avoid further stress, the patient may even tell the doctor that he is satisfied with the injections, but a detailed inquiry may reveal that he hardly, if ever, uses them.

The *doctor's attitude and personality* are critical factors for the development of a strong therapeutic alliance. In order to make this happen, the doctor must be genuinely encouraging and supportive of the patient's desire for a better sexual relationship with his partner. It is helpful if the couple senses the doctor's real delight in their sexual improvement. Therefore, he or she must be personally open and nonjudgmental about sex, and comfortable with inquiring into the couple's sexual behavior and experience in the minute detail necessary for the giving of effective instructions. Above all, the doctor must pay attention to and be empathic with the deeper emotional and sexual needs of both partners.

Methods of Administration

Some doctors administer a penile injection of papaverine or VIP and phentolamine to the patient in their offices and if this produces a good erection, they instruct the man to go home to his partner at once and to try to have intercourse with her before the erection abates (Zorgniotti & Lizza, 1987). Some practitioners who use this method do not bother to meet the wife; some go so far as to advise the patient to rent a hotel room in the vicinity of their offices and to have the partner waiting there.

This set-up is so stressful for most patients and for their partners that it guarantees the maximum incidence of noncompliance. For this reason, and because this is so disrespectful and so insensitive to patients' emotional needs, I strongly advise against this method of administration. No doubt this approach has led to successful outcomes in some cases. But I have seen numerous patients and couples, who eventually made an excellent adaptation to the pharmacologically induced erections, who were initially so turned off by this "Rush home and do it" approach that it took months (in one case, two years) for them to seek further help.

The first case of this kind, which I saw in 1987, is typical.

CASE 1.—NON-COMPLIANCE IN A MAN WITH ORGANIC IMPOTENCE*

Professor A, a 72-year-old diabetic mathematician with a history of progressive impotence, with his wife, age 59, consulted me with the hope that I would find the husband's erectile difficulties to be psychogenic and amenable to sexual therapy. Two months prior to the consultation, Professor A had been given an intrapenile injection of papaverine in a urologist's office on the assumption that he had diabetic impotence. This had produced a firm erection. Although Mrs. A knew nothing about this and although the doctor had never met her and had no

---

*This case has been reported in a previous publication (Kaplan, 1990c).

way of predicting her reactions, he instructed the patient to drive home with his erection as quickly as possible and to have intercourse with his wife before the erection abated.

Professor A, who was a sensitive, soft-spoken, shy, and mild-mannered man, tried to follow the doctor's instructions, albeit with much trepidation. He drove home with his erection and found that his wife was having a social gathering with some women friends. Concealing the bulge of his erection under some papers and with great embarrassment, he asked her to excuse herself and join him in the bedroom. When he showed her why he had summoned her, this emotionally fragile rejection-sensitive, phobically anxious woman burst into tears. She was offended by the mechanical, nonintimate manner in which she was being asked to participate in sex. Since that time, the couple had avoided sexual contact altogether.

The medical workup confirmed the primarily organic nature of this patient's impotence. This was evidenced by his abnormal NPT record, which showed only a single, brief tumescent episode over three consecutive nights of testing with a home monitor. In addition, the patient's glycohemoglobin was abnormally high, but his sex hormone levels were within normal limits. These findings were consistent with the clinical picture of erectile dysfunction in the presence of a normal libido.

I advised the couple that the husband's erectile difficulties were primarily organic and that, unfortunately, his erectile reserve was too limited to enable him to have intercourse, even under optimal emotional conditions and recognizing that A's potency problem did not reflect a lack or desire for his wife. Despite this, at their insistence I accepted the couple for a brief trial of sex therapy. We had five therapy sessions together during which we worked on reducing the husband' performance anxiety, improving the couple's techniques of physical stimulation, and resolving their resistance to exploring fantasy and erotica together.

At the same time, in the office sessions, I focused on helping Mrs. A overcome her irrational overreaction to her husband's erectile difficulties, which she took as a personal rejection (and blamed on his mother) despite all evidence to the contrary. This woman had a deep underlying fear of abandonment, which derived from her childhood, and the doctor's insensitive method of administrating pharmacotherapy had tapped into and further exaggerated her fears.

The couple were pleased by the increased emotional intimacy and physical closeness that resulted from their conjoint therapy sessions and from their "homework" exercises. They learned to enjoy mutual orgasms by oral and manual stimulation, and their anxieties about his erections diminished. However, even in this calmer emotional climate, A's erections were not sufficiently improved for intercourse and it became clear to them that if they wanted this, they would have to accept the injections.

It was only after Mrs. A's sense of security had improved to a point where she stopped personalizing her husband's diabetic impotence and no longer felt threatened by the "mechanical erections" that the couple were ready to accept the penile injections.

I worked with them for a few more sessions to help them integrate the injection-produced erections into their lovemaking in an intimate, emotionally reassuring manner, that would not threaten this emotionally vulnerable woman. Thus, they were advised that he should not inject himself prior to lovemaking. I suggested that they always start any sexual contact by commencing foreplay without the injection, and then turn to this only if both became sufficiently aroused, and only after he had communicated his desire to have intercourse with her, and while emphasizing that he was willing to forego sex if *she* did not wish this, and only after he had made it clear that he loved her and that he was not just using her for his sexual release.

Many persons would be put off by a woman's constant need for reassurance and declarations of love. But the reality is that this is what it takes to make a relationship work with a fragile, narcissistic partner; fortunately, Professor A rather liked the role.

On follow-up, one year later, the couple were having sex on a regular basis. Some of the time, they stimulated each other to climax orally or manually, without the injections, but occasionally they used the injection to have intercourse as a "special treat," mainly when *she* desired penetration.

While it is certainly possible that this emotionally fragile woman might have resisted her husband's using the injections even if this had been administered in a more private, sensitive manner, nevertheless the doctor's sending A home with a "prefabricated" erection that "had nothing to do with me" frightened her and made her feel defenseless. Her "irrelevance" in this situation was her nightmare come true, and this did not help her accept the injections.

I have since seen several patients who had negative reactions to this "rush-home" method of administration. One was a man with a severe obsessive-compulsive personality disorder who decompensated. He had a panic attack and became immobilized when he was about to leave the urologist's office fully erect in order to comply with his doctor's suggestion that he get into a taxi and go to his girlfriend's apartment across town. This patient needed intensive psychiatric care to recover from this episode.

This was an extreme example. Usually adversive psychiatric reactions resulting from inappropriate methods of administration are less severe. Other patients we have seen were typically only temporarily upset by the doctor's instructions that they go out in public with their erection and rush to their partners to try it out. And, not surprisingly, partners often object to this method also. Can you imagine what it feels like for a woman to wait like a prostitute in a hotel room in order to receive her partner with his new artificially induced erection that he wishes to test out on her? Hardly an occasion for intimacy and affection, nor is this approach designed to make the woman feel that she is important to her partner. Rather, she is apt to surmize that he is just using her to improve his ability to perform.

A more flexible approach that is sensitive to the patient's psychosexual needs, like the one described by Dr. Wagner in the preceding chapter, seems to work best from the standpoint of reducing the risks of noncompliance.

From a psychological point of view, we recommend that the patient receive a test dose in the physician's office so that it can be determined that this is effective and safe, how long the erection will last, and which mixture is appropriate for that particular patient. This gives the doctor the opportunity to observe the patient's physical and emotional reaction to the injections procedure and allows him to be there to support the patient and to respond to his questions and concerns.*

When the patient attains a satisfactory erection, and after he has learned to inject himself properly and is comfortable, and when it has been determined that the duration of the drug-induced tumescence will not be excessive, he can then be given a supply of the pre-mixed sterile solution of vasoactive material and syringes to use in the privacy of his home. There he can integrate the injection-induced erections into his love life at his own pace, and in ways that are compatible with his own individual emotional and sexual needs and those of his partner.

Many patients are initially anxious about injecting themselves into their genitalia. These fears are quite normal and they usually respond to the doctor's patient reassurance. But patients with underlying anxiety disorders can have severe reactions that require special attention.

One of my patients could not use the injections because he was phobic of needles; he actually experienced an episode of syncope. He was eventually able to inject himself successfully, but only after a careful, time-consuming process of systematic in-vivo desensitization to his needle phobia. The injections were initially given by the urologist**

---

*The method described above is possible only if the doctor's office is equipped for sterile repackaging of the medication. This should be a requirement for all clinicians treating patients with ICI.

**The urologist was Dr. Francois Eid, head of the pharmacologic injection program at the New York Hospital–Cornell Medical Center.

while the patient was lying down to prevent his passing out. When he became accustomed to this, he learned to inject himself, still in a supine position. No attempt was made to involve his partner until he felt entirely comfortable with the procedure.

Humane Instructions and Guidance

Physicians who administer pharmacologic injection programs tend to be meticulous and professional about the instructions they give regarding the medical aspects of this procedure. Thus, patients generally receive excellent advice and information about safe and effective techniques for injecting themselves, and about maintaining the sterility and the proper care and storage of their medication and syringes. But, important as this technical information surely is, by itself this is not enough to reduce the incidence of noncompliance because this does not consider the vital issue of patients' emotional needs (Kaplan, 1990).

Of course, it is important to teach the patient where to place the needle and how to push through the fascia so that the vasoactive material gets into the corpora. But it is just as important to ask him to discuss just exactly how he plans to use the injections when he goes home to his partner and how they both feel about this, as well as to correct any obvious errors and pitfalls. Sensitive psychological counseling that includes specific and detailed suggestions about how to introduce the injection procedure to his partner and how to make himself comfortable with the injections in the sexual situation can do much to forestall resistances and make the difference between compliance and noncompliance.

While there are many "wrong" ways to instruct patients with regard to using their injections, there is no one "right" way that will work in every case. People are simply too diverse in their cultural, sexual, and emotional needs, so it is not possible to devise a standard protocol that will be uniformly effective. However, the clinician can be guided by the following general principles:

1. The instructions the patient receives should be sensitive to his cultural values. For example, middle- and upper-class American couples (providing they have no major psychiatric problems or reservations about using the injections) are usually well advised not to use the injection unless they both feel desire. Therefore, I may suggest that they begin by engaging in foreplay in their usual manner. If both partners become aroused, and if they both agree that they want to have intercourse, the man is to excuse himself and go to the bathroom, where he injects himself. He then returns and the couple resume lovemaking. Both partners should be prepared for what to expect. They should know that the erection usually develops within five to ten minutes after injection, that the response is likely to be enhanced by erotic stimulation, and that they can make love slowly and gently, confident that the tumescence will last for about 30 to 40 minutes.

But not all cultures place as much emphasis on foreplay or on male-female mutuality as we do in the West, and the doctor should try not to impose his/her own values. To facilitate compliance in individuals from more male-oriented societies, it is often wiser to validate and help the man to maintain his image of dominance and virility. If this seems to be important in a particular case, I might suggest that the patient refrain from telling his partner about the injections, that he inject himself in privacy when he is ready to have sex, and that he fantasize and stimulate himself, on the assumption that he will feel less vulnerable if he approaches his partner only after he has already achieved an erection or at least when he senses that this is just about to develop.

2. *The instructions should also be tailored to fit the needs of the partner.* ICI programs are not likely to be successful if the partner is negative about the procedure. This can be a real problem.

Wives have various reactions to the husband's use of the injections. When these are negative, they can become powerful sources of resistance to the couple's successful adaptation. While some wives are eager for their husbands to have stronger erections and may actually insist that they use the injections when they make love, others strongly object to any evidence of artificial "love aids." The physician's taking such differences into account when he advises his patient about how to use the injections when he gets home can do much to forestall noncompliance. The following case vignettes illustrate a flexible approach to counseling that is individualized to accommodate the specific cultural, emotional, and sexual requirements of each case.

CASE 2.—MANAGING A DIFFICULT PARTNER

One of my patients, B, a 58-year-old diabetic attorney with progressive visual problems, had real difficulties getting his wife of 30 years to cooperate with the ICI program. Mrs. B was a beautiful woman, but she had a severe narcissistic personality disorder that prevented her from being able to empathize with her husband's suffering. She saw the problem strictly in terms of herself. She felt that she was being victimized by her husband's illness and she wanted nothing to remind her of this. She became especially upset when she was confronted with any evidence of the injections. She objected to his taking a rather long time in the bathroom to inject himself, completely ignoring the fact that he was handicapped by his poor eyesight. She would not let him keep his paraphernalia in the icebox, claiming that even if he hid this behind the eggs (which he tried to do) their teenage son might find it, which would be "unbearably" embarrassing for her.

His attempts to reason with her, reminding her that the family knew he had diabetes and needed injections, did not persuade her. At the same time, she insisted on intercourse, which of course he could not perform without the injections, as the only sexual option; she avoided his attempts to gratify her with oral or manual stimulation.

The presence of a personality disorder in the symptomatic patient or in the spouse is of bad prognostic significance for sex therapy as well as for ICI, because it is extremely difficult to engage such individuals in the therapeutic process, as was evidenced in this case.

This woman's narcissistic personality was a serious stumbling block to the couple's using the injections successfully. However, her husband's high motivation partially made up for this. Despite her total insensitivity to his needs and her almost bizarre level of self-involvement, this man was crazy about his wife and he was willing to go to any lengths to resume sex with her. This enabled us to work out an injection strategy that accommodated her narcissism, but did not stir up her underlying vulnerability.

First we *joined her resistance* to facing the fact that her husband was diabetic, losing his vision, and impotent. Towards this end, B was advised to hide all evidence of his illness and of the injections. He bought a small refrigerator, which he kept in his own bathroom for his medication, and he concealed the syringes in his office. Also, because there was some justification for her complaints that he was slow with his injections, I first had him practice injecting himself and masturbating in privacy, without involving her in the learning process. He did not approach her sexually until he had learned to inject himself more rapidly and until he was confident of his ability to perform with his injection-induced erections.

After he had accomplished this, they did make love, but rather infrequently, and not before he had performed some "special service" for her (such as scrubbing the bathroom thoroughly or driving downtown in the middle of the night for some special Chinese food). He would then inject himself surreptitiously and approach her, confident that the erection would develop. Sometimes, she would consent; at those times they would have surprisingly good and mutually enjoyable sex during which she was multiply orgastic.

This strategy was successful, at least partially, only because it accommodated the particular dynamics of this couple's relationship—her intractable narcissism and his need to serve, which bordered on the masochistic. But the couple required expert professional guidance in working this out.

3. The doctor must be flexible, and his suggestions should flow out of his understanding of the psychodynamics and the sexual needs of each individual whom he treats. Once again, there can be no set rules or recipes about how the partner should be involved in the injection program.

CASE 3.—CONCEALING THE USE OF INJECTIONS

Dr. C, a 76-year-old physician with advanced presbyrectia, was also advised to conceal his use of injections from his partner, but for very different psychological reasons. He was having a passionate affair with a young woman in her late twenties. Her fantasy and her image of him were that of a virile, powerful father-figure. He had a reciprocal fantasy of being the hero and mentor of an adoring young woman. He was afraid to tarnish his romantic image with the admission that he needed injections to function.

However, Dr. C was an extremely ethical and scrupulously honest man; thus, he felt guilty about withholding this information from her. In the therapy sessions, we worked through his underlying guilt about erotic pleasure and about having obtained his sexual fantasy. He came to see that revealing his impotence would only be destructive to the relationship and to their mutual sexual pleasure. This insight allowed him to conceal his injections and to enjoy his affair without guilt or conflict.

In other cases, the partner will feel left out if the patient takes sole responsibility for the injections. The procedure works much better for such couples if both partners are encouraged to participate actively in the injection process. Sometimes, the partner actually administers the injections.

CASE 4.—PARTNER-PROVIDED INJECTIONS

A 70-year-old homosexual man, D, was despondent about his progressively more severe organic impotence. His depression was heightened by the fact that he was about to go on a long-planned and eagerly anticipated trip with his lover, to celebrate his 70th birthday. Now he was disheartened by the prospect that there would be no sex. He was elated when I told him that he might find injection therapy helpful. He had a satisfactory response to an injection of papaverine in the urologist's office. However, his lover objected when he heard about this. He was a physician who lived in another part of the country where people regarded him as straight. He was able to see my patient only on rare occasions, during his holidays. The idea that during the months that they were apart D would be able to give himself an erection and have sex with anyone anytime he wanted to was threatening to his lover and he refused to cooperate.

My patient was eager to have sex, but he was also very hesitant about injecting himself; this proved to be the key to resolving the dilemma. Both were delighted with my suggestion that the doctor do the injecting and take responsibility for the paraphernalia. It was reassuring to the doctor to realize that his lover was too squeamish to inject himself and that the injections would be used only when he himself administered them. They had a wonderful birthday trip.

Another couple, heterosexuals, also used the strategy of partner-provided injections, but the dynamics were different.

The patient, who developed diabetic impotence at age 40, was an extremely good-looking, charming, but immature man, who was married to a strong-minded nursing supervisor who adored him and was very possessive of him.

The patient had a good response to intracavernosal injections of prostaglandin E_1 and phentolamine, and was given a sterile solution for home use. But the couple avoided using the injections to make love until they had worked out a routine, with the help of their therapist, that accommodated their interlocking emotional and sexual needs.

When the wife was in the mood to make love, she would signal her husband by leaving a syringe on his pillow. He felt great excitement at this sign of her affection. She would then skillfully inject him, while he lay on his back with his eyes closed, and then they would make love.

Both felt more comfortable when she was in control of their sexual relationship. He was most pleased by this scenario, which gratified his masochistic fantasies of being dominated by a powerful and nurturing woman. For her part, she loved being in charge of sex and in control of a handsome man.

THE PARTNER

Partner resistance and noncompliance is the single most common cause of treatment failure for all treatments for impotence, sex therapy as well as pharmacotherapy. In

other words, enlisting the partner's unqualified cooperation is a crucial ingredient in the successful adaptation to
and compliance with injection therapy programs. Thus,
it is well worth the doctor's time and effort to meet with
the partner, to get to know her, and to attempt to engage
her firmly into the treatment process. This can be accomplished only if she is addressed with the same interest,
empathy, and understanding that is extended to the symptomatic patient.

Sometimes, a wife is fully aware that she is ambivalent
about the injections or that she is resisting cooperating
because she is simply too angry at her husband. More
often than not, however, these insecurities and angers that
mobilize the partner's resistances operate on an unconscious level and the person has no insight into her sabotaging behavior.

Some women are threatened by the injections and sabotage them because they are afraid, consciously or unconsciously, that they will lose power and control in their
relationships when their husbands can have pharmacologic
erections and no longer depend on them sexually. Some
wives anticipate abandonment, fearing that their husbands
do not really love them, but stayed with them only because
they tolerated their sexual disability; they worry that their
men will have affairs with younger, more attractive partners once they regain their potency.

In most cases, these fears have no basis in reality. In
actual fact, partners often feel closer to each other and
more committed as a result of sharing this process. But for
women who are fundamentally insecure about their attractiveness as females, and for those who had poor sexual
relationships with their husbands prior to the onset of
their impotence, the husband's use of injections can tap

into the wife's preexisting feeling of low self-esteem and rekindle her latent separation problems. Under such circumstances, it is not surprising that the woman does not cooperate; in fact, she may try to discourage her husband's becoming comfortable with the injections.

Case 1, that of Professor A and his wife, was a good illustration of an insecure partner's sabotage. The second case illustrates a somewhat more complex, but basically similar dynamic. Such cases do not end successfully unless the wife can be convinced that the husband is appreciative of her efforts and that he is not solely interested in his own sexual gratification. Above all, if she is going to cooperate, she must trust that he is not going to turn to other women as soon as he has exploited her to become skillful at making love with the injections.

The husband's attempt to regain his potency with the injections can also stir up a wife's long-buried anger.

The following case is interesting in that it demonstrates clearly how the partner's attitude can make the difference between success and failure in adapting to the intracavernosal injections.

CASE 5.—UNCOOPERATIVE WIFE; COOPERATIVE MISTRESS*

The patient, E, was a 65-year-old retired army officer, who had avoided sex with his attractive wife for the past four years because he was experiencing increasing difficulty in attaining and maintaining erections. The medical workup revealed that he had moderate vasculogenic impotence.

---

*This case was briefly described in a previous publication (Kaplan, 1990c).

E was able to achieve a satisfactory erection after injection in the urologist's office and was given papaverine to be used at home. But he avoided any further sexual contact with his wife after the first disastrous attempt.

This couple had serious long-standing marital struggles that posed an obstacle to their resuming a sexual relationship. Although she was charming and superficially agreeable, this woman was brutally angry at her controlling, aggressive husband whose dominations she had helplessly endured for 25 years. His recent sexual disability created the perfect opportunity for her to get even, although she was totally unaware that she was acting out of pent-up anger.

When he came out of the bathroom with his injection-induced erection, ready to make love to her for the first time in years, she ridiculed and demeaned him. When he tried to have intercourse nevertheless, she criticized the way he touched her and kissed her and she was totally unresponsive. He managed to penetrate but did not ejaculate. The following evening, she rubbed salt in his wound by pointedly discussing the breakup of a marriage of a friend, a 70-year-old wealthy man and his glamorous 30-year-old second wife, by saying, "No wonder she needed a younger lover, I hear Bill couldn't get it up."

The patient, a proud and self-sufficient man who found it difficult to communicate with women, told me that he had been so humiliated by his wife's attacks on him that, without saying a word to her about how he felt, he had visited an old girlfriend. He had seen this woman on and off for the last 10 years. She was a warm and relaxed person, extremely fond of E, and

respectful and supportive and sensitive to his underlying vulnerability. She minimized his sexual difficulties and when he told her about the injections she
made a happy game of it: "Oh, we're going to have
so much fun together with your new weapon."
Despite his initial reservations about injecting himself,
with her loving supportive help he had no problem
having enjoyable intercourse.

SEXUAL HISTORY AND
SEXUAL STATUS

As was noted in Chapter III, the assessment of the
patient's sexual status is an essential part of the compre-
hensive evaluation of candidates for injection therapy.

The importance of the doctor's insight into his patient's
sexual desires and his concern for minimizing noncompliance have been a recurrent theme of this chapter. Conversely, many treatment failures can be attributed directly
to an inadequate sexual history, taken by an uninformed
and embarrassed physician. To avoid such errors, the doctor should not proceed with the injections until he has a
crystal-clear and detailed picture of the patient's current
sexual functioning and experience, as well as an understanding of the significant issues of his psychosexual
development.

Patients seldom volunteer the details of their sexual
experience to the doctor and this important information
must be actively elicited. However, once they are asked,
most people are quite forthcoming and often eager to air
their complaints, providing the physician's attitude is comfortable, helpful, and professional, and that he/she is

knowledgeable about and accepting of the infinite variety of human sexual behavior.

The patient tells you he is impotent. But that is hardly enough information. The details are very important for making an accurate diagnosis and for planning treatment. Can he get an erection at all? Under what circumstances? On oral sex? Or only when his partner expects to have intercourse? On masturbation? When there is no perform-ance pressure? In the A.M.? Nocturnally? With all part-ners? Does he mean that his penis does not get firm enough for penetration? Or does he have trouble staying erect? Under what circumstances does he lose his erection? When he is about to enter? During foreplay? When he is giving his partner oral stimulation? In the vagina? What does he think of when he is engaging in sex? Is he worried about his erection? Coming too fast? Do extraneous thoughts intrude?

It is also important to ascertain the patient's level of desire and any changes in his ejaculatory sensations and control. Is he attracted to his partner? Does he climax too rapidly? Is this new? Or does it take too long to come? Does it hurt? How does he feel after he comes?

It is also important to determine how well the patient functioned prior to the onset of his potency problems. (If he functioned well, the prognosis is generally favorable.) How frequently did he have sex? Did he have any prob-lems? What kind? Was his ejaculatory control adequate or a source of concern? How strong was his desire?

Did the patient experience any childhood sexual trauma? Incest? Rape? What were the "sexual messages" he received during his childhood? Was sex regarded as dirty? Dangerous? Sinful? OK? Is his attitude about sex strictly moralistic? (This can be a source of problems.) Libertarian? What is his masturbation history? Is he free or guilty about self-stimulation? What are his sexual fantasies? What are his attitudes about erotica and sexual fantasy? Does he feel guilty about using injections to enhance his sexual pleasure?

Without such detailed information, serious errors in management can occur and may undermine the doctor-patient relationship and the success of treatment.

For example, some physicians have their patients view erotic videotapes in their offices when they are testing out the efficacy of the injections. This can be very useful. Focusing on erotica serves to distract the patient from his fears and also adds a dimension of psychic stimulation that can act in synergy with the vasoactive medication.

But the doctor should know this would pose problems for his orthodox Jewish or devout Roman Catholic patients, who are not allowed to look at erotica nor to engage in sexual fantasy, as these acts are considered by these religious denominations to be major sins against God.

It is also important for the doctor to gain some insight into the patient's sexual relationship with his partner, and gain a picture of her sexual functioning and her feelings about the injection program. Do they love each other? (If so, you can count on cooperation.) Are there problems in the relationship? (These can prevent her from a full commitment to the treatment program.) Is she attracted to him? Does she enjoy sex? Is she orgastic? Does she have a sexual problem that may interfere with compliance? What kind? Is she anxious about sex? Prudish? Is she a good sexual partner? Is she postmenopausal? Does she lubricate? Is she receiving estrogen replacement? How does she react when her partner loses his erection? Is she supportive? Does she take it personally? How does she feel about her partner using the ICIs? Happy? Threatened? Angry? Neutral?

Dr. Wagner describes an elderly man he saw in consultation. This patient had been a good responder in the doctor's office, but he continued to complain to the urologist, "It doesn't work" (at home) even after the dosage of the vasoactive drug had been increased. When Dr. Wagner took a detailed sexual history, it turned out that the man's erections were fine. The trouble was that his elderly wife had severe atrophic vaginitis and simply couldn't tolerate penetration. The urologist had not thought to inquire about the partner.

SEXUAL DESIRE DISORDERS

Prior to commencing ICI, it is essential to establish the status of the patient's libido, because a lack of sexual desire on the part of the patient and/or the partner is a major cause for noncompliance and/or for failure to use the penile injections successfully.

When a person has no desire to make love to the partner or, worse still, if either is actually repelled by the other, the likelihood of successful adaptation to ICI is very low. It is very difficult for a woman who loathes her husband's touch to be the encouraging and enthusiastic partner he needs while he is struggling to learn to use the injections. Similarly, the man who finds his wife's personality unpleasant and her body physically unattractive, and who is having sex only out of a sense of obligation, is likely to resent and to resist having to inject himself into his penis in order to be able to have a sexual experience he does not really want.

A certain level of desire is necessary for a couple to enjoy lovemaking, with or without the injections. Without any passion or lust, the sexual experience is apt to be mechanical and devoid of pleasure; eventually, sex may become an unpleasant experience.

Two axes of sexual desire are significant from a clinical perspective: one is the *intensity,* the other is deficiency of desire, if the latter is a problem, it is important to ascertain whether this is *global* or *specific* to the partner.

Sexual desire is a subjective feeling, described as lust or horniness or a hunger for sex, that moves the individual to seek out and/or to respond to sexual stimulation. A state of aroused sexual desire also heightens the pleasure of genital functioning.

The magnitude of sexual desire may be conceptualized as lying on a continuum:

1. Hypersexuality (Don Juanism, nymphomania) occupies the highest point on this continuum. This is a pathological con-

TABLE VI.1
Continuum of Sexual Desire

	DESIRE STATE	DIAGNOSIS
1	Hyperactive Desire	Sexual addiction Nymphomania Don Juanism
2	Spontaneous Desire	Normal
3	Desire easily evoked	Normal
4	Desire difficult to evoke	Hypoactive desire (HSD)
5	Desire cannot be evoked	Hypoactive desire (HSD)
6	Active dislike of sex	Sexual aversion Phobic avoidance of sex

dition where the sex drive is so urgent that it interferes with the person's functioning. The "sexual addict" or the compulsively sexual individual is interested in little else but having sex as frequently as possible, to the neglect of work and family.

The notion of sexual addiction has become quite popular in the U.S. However, it is not clear if hypersexuality or sexual addiction is a real phenomenon. The DSM-III-R subcommittee on sexual dysfunctions reviewed the diagnostic criteria of desire disorders; it was concluded that there was insufficient evidence to warrant including this diagnostic category into the nomenclature. To be sure, there are people who are compulsive about and preoccupied with sex. But the question was raised that the term "sexual addiction" might simply be evidence of the New Puritanism, which seems to be emerging, and that it might be a disservice to people with a high sex drive to label them as "sexual addicts" or as pathologically hypersexual.

Sexually hyperactive individuals are extremely compliant with ICI. In fact, these are the patients who may compulsively overuse the injections to the point of harming themselves.

One of my diabetic patients, a widower who was obsessed with women and extremely compulsive sexually, persisted in using the injections (of which he had a large supply) five or six times a week, sometimes twice in one evening, even though he had been warned by his urologist to stop because he was developing penile nodules.

2. Spontaneous desire. Under normal circumstances, desire arises spontaneously after a period of abstinence, at least in younger males. Spontaneous desire is less common in older men and also in women, who are often highly responsive to sexual stimulation but do not experience sexual frustration in the absence of a partner. (There is some evidence that this gender difference might be changing in our society.) Sexual desire also arises spontaneously in men and in women when they are in love, and especially when they are near the object of their desire.

3. Responsive desire. Next on the libido scale are individuals whose desire is easily aroused by the partner or by extraneous erotic stimulation, but who do not feel spontaneous desire. These individuals, as well as those with a spontaneously fluctuating sex hunger, are considered entirely normal and their prognosis for the successful use of ICI is good (providing of course that there are no other psychological obstacles).

4. Hypoactive sexual desire. The next two levels of sexual desire are considered to be pathological and are classified in DSM-III-R under the category Inhibited Sexual Desire (ISD), and will be termed hypoactive sexual desire (HSD) in DSM-IV. (APA, 1980, 1992). Men afflicted by this syndrome have great difficulty in becoming aroused; those with severe forms of ISD cannot get excited at all, no matter what type of erotic stimulation they employ. Patients with deficient sexual desire are often conflicted about wanting to have sex with their partner. These men tend to avoid sex, whether they can have erections or not, and they are often noncompliant with ICI.

5. Sexual aversion. The most extreme sexual desire disorder is an active sexual aversion or the phobic avoidance of sex. These men, who are terrified or repelled by sex with any and all partners, have a very poor prognosis with

ICI. The following case vignette illustrates a treatment failure in a man who could not overcome his sexual aversion to his wife.

CASE 6.—SEXUAL AVERSION, TREATMENT FAILURE

The couple, a 45-year-old man and his 36-year-old wife, were well-to-do East Indian Moslems. They had been married for 12 years and had six children, all girls. They consulted me because Mrs. F was obsessed with becoming pregnant again, as she desperately wanted a boy, but Mr. F had become impotent.

The couple had an extremely combative relationship. A handsome man, F was cold, aloof, and controlling, while she was obese, and extremely angry at him. Although he was ambivalent about having another child and was not attracted to his wife, he felt it was the right thing to do and he tried to comply. F avoided sex with his wife except during her fertile periods. However, when he did attempt intercourse with her at these times, he was unable to attain an erection.

The couple wanted ICI in order to resolve the problem, but although the patient had excellent erections in response to intracavernosal injections of papaverine, this case was a treatment failure.

F's ambivalence about being 'used" for reproduction by a woman he found unattractive physically and whose personality he detested was manifested in his multiple resistances. He missed several appointments with his urologist because he "forgot." On several of the nights he was supposed to have sex with his wife, he managed to have urgent business meetings. He also developed disabling migraine headaches, which occurred mostly on weekends. In response to her husband's continued avoidance of sex, despite the fact that it was clear that if he *wanted* to he *could* have erections with the injections, Mrs. F became angrier and angrier. This couple's hostilities escalated to the point where she would constantly berate him as soon as he entered the house; as a result, he spent less and less time at home.

It was not possible for me to resolve this couple's anger at each other and their resistances to sex. Since in their culture divorce was out of the question, the F's continued to live together in a state of "cold war," without any sexual contact.

Biological Aspects of Sexual Desire

The attempt to override serious psychogenic inhibitions of sexual desire by means of penile injections is not only likely to fail but can actually be psychiatrically hazardous. However, the prognosis is much better when the loss of sexual desire is due to physical causes, because these men are not ambivalent about sex.

The experience of sexual desire is more than a mental or cognitive event. It is the product of a biologically based drive state that depends on the activation of the sex regulatory centers of the brain (Kaplan, 1979, McEwen et. al, 1979). Certain disease states and drugs can impair the sex drive on a physical basis. These include drugs that depress the sex centers directly and medical conditions that interfere with the production and bio-availability of testosterone or the overproduction of prolactin (Kaplan, 1979, 1983; Seagraves, 1988, 1990). Therefore, when a patient has lost his sexual desire globally, that is in all circumstances—for his partner, for fantasy, for other partners, for masturbation—one must rule out organic causes in order to detect potentially correctable physical problems prior to commencing with ICI.* In contrast to men with psychogenic desire disorders, patients with physical problems may be excellent candidates for ICI. Although the injections provide only mechanical erections and do not increase sexual feelings, these men and their partners are often conflict-free about using the injections to resume sexual intercourse.

For example, I have seen two patients with prostate cancer who had lost their capacity to experience sexual desire because of low testosterone levels—brought about in one case by castration and in the other by anti-androgen therapy. In both cases, the men were delighted to be able to provide sexual gratification for their wives, and the women saw this as a sign of their husband's love. Not surprisingly, these couples made excellent adaptations to the injections, even though these cancer patients could no longer feel sexual passion. The restoration of potency actually had a beneficial effect on the self-esteem of these cancer patients, while also bringing the couples closer emotionally.

MANAGING RESISTANCE TO ICI

The brief, active, psychodynamically oriented therapy that was originally developed to overcome the resistances of patients with psychogenic impotence to the process and

---

*Our endocrine workup for the loss of sexual desire and impotence in males includes testosterone, free testosterone, DEA, prolactin, LH, FSH, estradiole and glycohemoglobin. When indicated, we also include a thyroid profile and, in older men, growth hormone (Kaplan, 1983).

the outcome of sex therapy (see Chapter VII) can often be effective in helping overcome noncompliance to ICI. When dealing with patients who are having trouble using their injections, we do not try to psychoanalyze them, even if they clearly have considerable emotional and/or marital problems. Rather, we focus only on helping the patient adapt successfully to the ICI and attempt to "bypass" any of the deeper problems that may have spawned his resistances to having a better sex life.

To implement this objective, we follow a systematic sequence of progressively "deeper" interventions when we encounter resistances to ICI, until the therapeutic impasse is resolved.

More specifically, when a patient shows signs of noncompliance—for example, not using his injections, or using them ineffectively, or creating difficulties with his partner, or approaching her at an inopportune moment—we offer him support and ask him to *repeat* his efforts to use the injections during the next week.

If the patient continues to avoid using the injections, we assume that something about the procedure is too threatening for him and we attempt to modify the circumstances under which he uses the injections so as to *reduce* the emotional impact of the procedure.

For example, an excessive need to please the partner is a frequent source of noncompliance in men with excessive rejection sensitivity. These men are so afraid that something will go wrong with the injections and that their partner will be displeased that they become too fearful to try it at all. In such cases, it is often helpful to advise the patient to "practice by himself"—to masturbate with a pharmacologically induced erection until he is comfortable enough with the procedure to risk approaching his partner.

Other patients need still more extensive psychological preparation before they can benefit from ICI.

One of my patients, a 25-year-old man with diabetic impotence, who attained excellent erections by injecting himself when alone, was too terrified to use these to make love to his fiancee. However, she insisted on this before she would marry him.

This young man was totally inexperienced and much too anxious about sex for the injections to make sense. He first needed to learn, with the help of his therapist and the cooperation of his fiancee, how to kiss, caress, stimulate, and be comfortable sexually with his partner before there could be any thought of intercourse, with or without the ICIs.

It has already been mentioned that partner-administered injections can help overcome the avoidance of certain patients who are afraid or unable (because of poor vision, tremors, etc.) to administer the injections to themselves. But once again, effective therapeutic strategies must flow out of the doctor's understanding of the couple's dynamics and of their sexual needs. Partner-provided injections will work only if the doctor makes certain that this will not make the wife see her husband as a sexual cripple.

Cognitive Restructuring

The *cognitive restructuring* of the sexual situation and of the injections so that these will be less threatening is another effective brief therapy maneuver. For example, one of my patients, a bachelor who was a diabetic, was ambivalent about and avoided using the injections to make love to his girlfriend because, in the mind of this highly ethical man, if he accepted her help in solving his sexual problems and if he had intercourse with her, he would feel obliged to acquiesce to her wish to get married.

The reality was that this highly neurotic young woman would have made a terrible long-term partner for him and that both would have been miserable in what could have been a most ill-conceived marriage. But she was a gorgeous woman who loved sex and she also loved going to the fine restaurants and taking the luxurious trips that my patient was happy to provide.

With the help of therapy, the patient was able to move away from the old "rule" that came from a highly moralistic upbringing, that if you sleep with a woman you must marry her, and he was also able to redefine consensual sex in a more adult way, as a mutually pleasurable experience, like a beautiful dance that both partners enjoy. And when he came to see that a long-term commitment was a separate issue, he felt freer to enjoy the benefits of the ICIs to make love.

Insight

Many of the patients we have seen have been helped to overcome their resistances and to make excellent adjustments to ICI in response to the kinds of brief behavioral and cognitive strategies described above, without needing to gain insight into their deeper problems.

But some patients are too deeply conflicted about sex

and about their partners to respond to such brief "super-ficial" tactics. Such patients usually have no awareness that they are sabotaging themselves, and they must be confronted with their self-destructive behavior before they can be engaged in the exploratory process that will lead them to a better sex life.

I often say to a patient who continues to botch up his injection program: "part of you certainly wants a better sex life. You went to all this expense and trouble and time. But another part of you seems to be sabotaging your efforts. It has been 10 weeks now and you always manage to find an excuse or make some mistake, and you have not yet had sexual intercourse with your injections although you certainly get wonderful erections. I'm afraid the negative part is winning, because last week when you were about to finally make love to your partner, you managed to have a big fight and she walked out."

Men with deeper self-destructive tendencies seldom improve sexually, unless they gain some insights into their unconscious conflicts about sex and into the childhood roots of these conflicts. With such patients, it is necessary to shift into a psychodynamic mode in order to help them overcome their sexual self-sabotage.

Unfortunately, psychological therapy, no matter how astute, will not help every patient. The following case illustrates a treatment failure.

CASE 7.—A TREATMENT FAILURE

Mr. G was a 58-year-old CEO of a large public company. He had recently developed impotence with his wife. He could still ejaculate while she fellated or manually stimulated him, but when he attempted to penetrate, he invariably lost his erection. His wife was extremely upset about this and for this reason the internist had referred G to a urologist for a trial of ICI. G found the procedure upsetting and could not bring himself to use the injections with his wife. Because of this and his wife's increasing agitation, the patient was referred to me for psychological treatment of his noncompliance.

It turned out that this caring, responsible man was very attached emotionally to his wife and his family, but he had absolutely no sexual interest in her. He was put off by her obesity (she weighed 300 lbs.). But this made him uncomfortable as he "bought" her position of refusing to diet on the grounds that "If you loved me, you'd love me as I am. Besides, if I lost 50 pounds, you would still be impotent." The patient also suffered from his wife's frequent mood swings, during which he became the target for her anger and depressions.

By contrast, this patient had functioned well with an extramarital partner. Although his erections had softened somewhat in recent years, he had been extremely attracted to this woman and his passion helped him compensate. He continued to function with her until the relationship ended several months ago. For obvious reasons, this level of performance was not possible with his wife.

This man was torn between his guilt about upsetting his wife by rejecting her and his reluctance to use the injections. He found it difficult to admit to himself that there were good reasons for his lack of desire, for his envy of his friends who all seemed to have more attractive and more pleasant wives, and for his ambivalence about forcing himself to make love to her. He was even more defensive against acknowledging that *she* had some responsibility for their sexual problem.

In this case, it was necessary for the patient to gain some insight into the unconscious transference he had made between his wife and his mother. His relationship with his mother, who had been widowed when the patient was 10, was characterized by his guilty and compulsive compliance with any and all of her wishes. To this day, he had never been able to say no to her. G began to realize that as his wife became increasingly heavier, she reminded him more and more of his mother, who had also been obese. This insight led him to a more realistic appraisal of his sexuality and of his marriage.

This case was a success in terms of the patient's feeling better about himself and attaining some insight, but it was a failure in that he resolved not to use the injections to have intercourse with his wife. In other words, this couple's problems were too complex to lend themselves to a mechanical solution. Fortunately, I was able to persuade this couple to enter long-term marital therapy to try to solve their considerable interpersonal difficulties as a prerequisite to improving their sexual relationship.

DETECTING PSYCHOPATHOLOGY

Once again, I cannot overemphasize that impotence and its treatments are highly charged emotionally, and that patients typically feel vulnerable and exposed, much more so than in response to other disease states or other medical procedures. Even stable patients in good marriages can have some problems adjusting to the injections. But individuals with meager psychological reserves are especially likely to have difficulties in benefiting from this treatment, no matter how sensitive and supportive the doctor is. Worse still, those with latent psychiatric disorders may react adversely to intrapenile injections—with depression, panic, paranoia, or obsessional states—and the treatment may even precipitate litigious attacks upon the doctor.

I do not think it necessary to conduct a complete psychiatric examination of every patient who seeks pharmacotherapy. However, for the reasons mentioned above, it is good medicine to include a brief psychiatric screening as part of the assessment of candidates for injection programs. It is especially important to screen out patients who are psychotic or suicidal. It is also wise to identify men with obsessive-compulsive personality disorders, anxiety disorders, and paranoid states, as well as those with serious problems relating to women who are in problematic relationships. Patients with these problems have a high risk of getting into emotional trouble with this treatment. The clinician should also be alert to partner pathology, especially looking for partners who are narcissistic or have severe separation problems, because such women are likely to sabotage their partner's injection therapy and will need careful management.

If a brief review of the patient's psychiatric history or his manner suggest the possibility of significant psychopathology, a psychiatric consultation is in order, preferably with a professional who has expertise in human sexuality, prior to instituting injection treatment.

That is not to say that psychiatric disorders, except for

acutely disturbed patients, constitute an absolute contra-indication to injection treatment. To the contrary, many men who have psychological problems eventually do very well with ICI even if they initially resist. In fact, in some cases the enhanced ability to function sexually that is provided by the injections can improve their self-esteem and their romantic relationships.

However, patients with certain neurotic problems may not be able to handle inserting a hypodermic needle into their phallus because, on a symbolic level, this can tap into old childhood fears and stir up their latent sexual anxieties and defenses.* Others who are shaky about their masculinity may overuse the injections compulsively, to a point where they hurt themselves physically or harm their relationships by pressuring their partners for sex. Such neurotic patients may eventually make excellent adjustments to penile injection therapy, but they tend to need professional help to prepare the way.

Unfortunately, I cannot say that every paranoid or compulsive or phobic patient can be successfully treated with injections, even with good psychiatric support. A certain number of psychiatrically related treatment failures will always occur. But this can be kept to a minimum if the injection treatment is combined with psychosexual therapy when this is indicated.

I have emphasized the psychiatric aspects of injection therapy in this chapter because this important issue has been neglected. But I do not mean to imply that every candidate for injection treatment needs or should have sexual

---

*According to Freudian theory, neurotic men who have not solved their childhood struggles with their parents unconsciously see sex as an incestuous act and carry a deeply buried fear that they will be killed or punished by castration.

therapy. Stable men with a negative psychiatric history who have functioned well prior to the onset of their erectile disorders and who are in harmonious marriages do not require adjuvant psychiatric treatment. It suffices if the physician who administers the injections is reasonably sensitive and caring. But neurotic patients are just as likely to develop diabetic impotence or impairment of their penile circulation as are those who enjoy robust mental health. Such patients with associated psychiatric conditions or preexisting sexual or marital problems often do much better with psychiatric assistance.

CHAPTER VII

Injection Treatment
for Older Patients

by Helen Singer Kaplan

IT IS WIDELY BELIEVED that getting older entails the loss of sexuality and that people lose their interest in sex as they age. But those are myths. In actual fact, sex is one of the last biological functions to fall prey to the aging process. There are countless older people who are wearing hearing aids or reading glasses or pacemakers, and there are even some who are confined to wheelchairs, who are still enjoying making love. Moreover, sexuality continues to be highly valued by many senior citizens and the loss of potency can be devastating to the aging man and to his partner. For these reasons, physicians should extend their best efforts to ameliorate impotence in their older patients.

SEX AND THE AGING PROCESS

A number of surveys of sexual behavior in the aging population have been conducted in the recent years (Kinsey et al., 1948, 1953; Palmore, 1970, 1974; George & Weiler, 1981; Starr & Weiner, 1981; Brecher, 1984; Todarello & Boscia, 1985; Weitzman & Hart, 1987). These studies,

TABLE VII.1
Sex and the Aging Process: Summary of Recent Studies

Study	Year	N	Age Range	Outcome
1. Kinsey Reports	1948 1953	212 ♂ 152 ♀ Σ 364	51–90 51–80	70 percent of couples are sexually active at age 70 on a regular basis. The average frequency over 70 is 0.3 times a week.
2. Masters and Johnson	1966 1970	150 ♂ 212 ♀ Σ 362	50–90	Found men and women in all age groups who remain sexually active on a regular basis.
3. Duke University Longitudinal Study	1953– 1965 1968– present	250 ♂ + ♀ 502 ♂ + ♀ Σ 752	60–90 45–69	70 percent of physically healthy couples have regular intercourse at the age of 68. In some cases, the frequency of sexual intercourse increases.
4. Starr-Weiner Report on Sex and Sexuality in the Mature Years	1981	280 ♂ 520 ♂ Σ 800	60–91	80 percent of total sample (♂ & ♀) are sexually active. 50 percent have sex on a regular basis. Of these, 50 percent have intercourse once a week or more often.
5. Consumer Union Survey: Love, Sex and Aging	1984	4,200 ♂ + ♀	50–93	79 percent of men, and 65 percent of women aged 70–91 are sexually active on a regular basis. 58 percent ♂ and 50 percent ♀ have sex every week.
All Studies Combined	1948– present	6,478 ♂ + ♀	50–93	The majority of physically healthy men and women remain sexually active on a regular basis into the 9th decade.

which involved thousands of men and women between the ages of 50 and 100, are unanimous in their findings that the majority of healthy older people remain sexually active on a regular basis into advanced old age. According to all studies conducted to date, close to 70 percent of men and women who are free of disease and are not taking medications with sexual side effects have sex about once a week when they are in their seventies (see Table VII.1)

I am not suggesting that men retain their youthful potency throughout life. There are, of course, certain inevitable age-related biological changes in male sexuality. In some cases, these lead to total impotence. In most cases, however, the aging process produces only partial deficits and the older man must adapt to these in order to remain functional (Kaplan, 1980, 1990b).

The aging process does not result in a general decline of the male sexual response, but has specific and different effects on the three phases of the male sexual response cycle: desire, excitement, and orgasm. It is important for the clinician who cares for older patients to be aware of these normal age-related biological changes and to understand the impact that these have on sexual behavior and functioning. The following is a summary of the normal age-related biological changes in males' sexual desire, excitement, and orgasm that have particular clinical significance in that these frequently play an important role in the pathogenesis of sexual complaints in older men (also see Table VII.2).

Desire

The male sex drive peaks at age 17 and thereafter gradually declines. After the age of 50, the effects of aging are

TABLE VII.2
The Effects of Age on Sexuality

PHASE	MALE		FEMALE	
I. Orgasm	A.	Significantly lengthened refractory period	A.	No significant effects
	B.	Decreased volume of ejaculate		
II. Excitement	A.	Erections are less firm	A.	Postmenopausal vaginal dryness and atrophy—caused by estrogen deficiency
	B.	Older men require increased and concomitant physical and mental stimulation in order to attain and maintain an erection		
	C.	Ability to maintain erection is decreased	B.	Vaginal laxness caused by cystocoele and rectocoele in parous women
	D.	Erections are more vulnerable to emotions and stress		
	E.	Paradoxical refractory period		
III Desire	A.	Variable—Some men and women maintain sexual desire into their 80s and 90s. Sex drive of others declines in the menopausal years—testosterone is a factor for both genders.		

highly variable and thought to be related, at least in part, to testosterone. Some men maintain a youthful level of androgens and sexual activity into advanced old age, while in others testosterone production begins to decline significantly when they reach their middle years. It is believed by some authorities that the resulting androgen-deficiency syndrome produces a significant loss of libido in older men, which has been termed the "male menopause." However, other experts doubt that this is a real phenomenon.

Injection therapy will do little to improve the sex lives of men whose complaints are the product of endocrine problems, except to provide them with mechanical tumescent episodes. When this is medically prudent, men whose erectile difficulties are secondary to demonstrable hormone deficiency states should be treated with hormone replacement and not with injections (Sciavi, 1976; Seagraves, 1988).

Erection

There is now increasing evidence that certain functional and morphological changes in penile anatomy and physiology can be related to age. More specifically, the volume percentage of smooth muscle is reduced by more than 25 percent from the age of 30 to 80 (Meuleman et al., 1990). In younger men, about 65 percent of the cell mass of the cavernous bodies is smooth muscle tissue and the rest connective tissue, which means that concerted interaction between cells is diminished and that compliance and elasticity are reduced as the older man loses penile muscle mass. Moreover, recent studies have indicated a significant age-dependent increase in tension development when the contracting agent phenylephrine was added to an organ bath with human tissue. This might imply that older men could have a higher "tone" of the smooth muscle if the same amount of adrenergic substance is present, thereby counteracting the relaxation necessary for full erection (Christ et al., 1990). This finding may also account, at least partially, for older men's greater vulnerability to the effects of the adrenergic surge that accompanies emotional stress on their erectile functioning (see Table VII.2).

With increasing age, especially after 40, sensitivity to vibratory and tactile stimuli decreases (Weiss, 1971).

In a group of older men, penile rigidity produced by

vibrators was compared with that produced by intercourse and a close positive correlation was found between age and penile rigidity (Newman, 1970). In practical terms this means that the same stimulation will evoke a reduced erectile response in an elderly man.

These new data provide the physical basis for the observation, which grew out of our clinical experience of working with older patients, that as a man ages he becomes progressively more dependent on his partner for increased erotic stimulation and emotional support in order to remain functional (Kaplan, 1980, 1990a, 1991).

The normal age-related changes in penile erection have been termed *presbyrectia* (Kaplan, 1989b) to distinguish these from the effect of certain disease states and drugs that have similar deleterious effects on the erectile response. The following five changes in erectile functioning are clinically important in the pathogenesis of impotence and sexual avoidance in older men:

1. Erections become less firm but, providing the partner is cooperative, remain rigid enough for penetration in most men into advanced old age.
2. When they are young, men are able to erect in response to physical stimulation of the genitalia or by psychic stimulation alone. As they get older, the capacity for spontaneous erection declines and penile sensitivity decreases. As a result, older men need progressively more intense physical stimulation and concomitant psychic erotic stimulation in order to achieve and maintain their erections.
3. The length of time an erection can be maintained decreases with age. If an older man makes too

much of an effort to hold back his ejaculation until his partner is satisfied, as he was able to do without difficulties in the past, he may develop potency problems on that account.

4. Erections become progressively more vulnerable to the physiological concomitants of emotional stress, especially to the adrenergic component.

5. Some men as they age experience a progressively longer delay in their ability to regain a lost erection even when they do not ejaculate. This has been called the "paradoxical refractory period" by Masters and Johnson (1970).

Orgasm

The refractory period, the length of time that must elapse after a man has ejaculated before he can be stimulated to another climax (when he is *refractory* to further sexual stimulation) increases substantially with age. This interval lengthens from just a few minutes at the age of 17 to as much as 48 hours or more by the age of 70. If the older man does not realize that this is a normal phenomenon, the fear that he is losing his sexuality can precipitate a secondary potency problem.

In sum, the male sexual response does not disappear with age, although it changes in significant ways. The ultimate result of these changes is to make men more dependent on women physically and emotionally. More specifically, as the aging male loses his ability to have spontaneous erections and his penile sensitivity lessens, he needs his partners to supply him with the additional physical stimulation of genitalia that he now requires to attain and maintain his erection. Furthermore, since his ability to function becomes increasingly vulnerable to the effects of the adrenergic surge that accompanies the experience of anxiety, the older man also becomes more dependent on his partner's unqualified emotional support and her acceptance of his current level of functioning.

Age and Female Sexuality

If the older man's partner is postmenopausal, she too faces age-related changes in her sexuality that can affect her husband's potency. While a woman's sex drive may not diminish appreciably after menopause and her ability to have orgasms often remains unchanged, she loses the bloom of her youthful physical attractiveness and must compensate for this with attractive personal qualities in order to remain an effective sexual partner. Moreover, postmenopausal women who do not receive hormone replacement develop estrogen-deficiency syndrome, which is characterized by atrophic changes of the female genitalia.

More specifically, the vagina loses its ability to lubricate in response to physical stimulation and tends to become dry and tight, as well as losing some of its erotic aroma, so that lovemaking often becomes painful (Wagner, 1986). These changes make lovemaking less exciting and intromission more difficult for their partners. Women who have borne children may develop a different problem. Multiparous women often suffer from a loss of vaginal muscle tone and a stretching of the introitus, with the result that their partners feel less penile stimulation on coital thrusting and may experience erectile difficulties on that account.

ADAPTATION VERSUS DYSFUNCTION

Our work with more than 500 patients with sexual complaints who were 50 years or older has made it clear that men who are able to adapt to their age-related physical impairments and couples who are able to maintain their sexual functioning despite these changes share a number of characteristics. For one, they enjoy harmonious, intimate, communicative relationships that include a commitment to each other's well-being and sexual pleasure. Two, the men are free enough of sexual and neurotic conflicts and enjoy sufficient self-esteem to feel entitled to good sex. And three, these couples are flexible and nonjudgmental in their sexual attitudes (Kaplan, 1990a, 1991).

Such loving older couples, who are conflict-free about sexual pleasure and highly committed and creative in their efforts to remain sexually active successfully, adapt to these age-related changes in the husband's erectile responses intuitively and imperceptibly. They accept his presbyrectia in the same constructive spirit as their presbyopia or their presbycussis as a natural part of getting older, without overreacting and without blaming their partners. Although his erections are a little softer, while her vagina is a little dryer, these intimate couples do not avoid sex. They are secure enough sexually and trust each other sufficiently to risk an occasional "failure."

The wife agrees, without making a power struggle out of it (although this may not be her first preference) to have sex in the morning when her elderly husband's erectile capacity is at its peak.

She does not take the absence of his spontaneous erections during foreplay as a personal rejection or as a sign that he is becoming impotent; rather, she lovingly supplies him, without being asked, with more intense penile stimulation. She may try oral or manual techniques to help his erections. Rather than objecting, she encourages his use of erotica (if this is compatible with the couple's value system) and she uses lubricants (prior to getting into bed with him so as not to create a stressful interruption) to protect her more fragile genitalia and to make penetration easier for him.

If the woman's vagina is lax,* the couple uses sexual techniques that heighten penile stimulation. These include using concomitant manual stimulation of the penis during intercourse and coital positions during which the woman closes her legs to provide additional friction to her partner's penis with her thighs. The man accepts these age-related changes of his wife's genitalia and accommodates to them without negative comment, while she is equally accepting of her aging partner's diminishing "staying power."

He, also without being asked, takes more time with foreplay and concentrates on giving his partner pleasure with manual and oral stimulation of her genitalia, to compensate for the briefer periods of vaginal penetration. He is extra-attentive to his postmenopausal wife, and makes sure to make her feel that she is still an attractive woman. And his thoughtfulness in turn inspires her to do her best to help him compensate for his presbyrectic changes.

Above all, sensing his increased vulnerability to emotional stress, she never threatens him with inappropriate performance demands, or with criticisms or negative com-

---

*Surgical repair of cystocoele and rectocoele is a relatively simple procedure and a good option for women with severe vaginal stretching.

ments about his virility, potency, or attractiveness. Older men who enjoy such flexible sexual attitudes and who are blessed with supportive partners can remain sexually active in the face of considerable biological deficit.

However, if the physical slowdown occurs in a setting of latent marital hostility, or if the couple is inflexible in their sexual behavior because of their culturally programmed sexual inhibitions, serious and chronic potency problems can develop in men who have only relatively minor organic changes.

ASSESSING PHYSICAL LIMITATIONS AND RESERVES

The medical evaluation of the impotent patient has been discussed by Dr. Wagner in Chapter III. A meticulous search for physical causes, especially for those that are reversible, is especially important in older men because the incidence of medical problems increases substantially as men age. Actually, if they receive a proper workup, about 50 percent of men who are 50 years or older are found to have some demonstrable physical impairments of their erectile response, which can be attributed to medications or disease states that affect their sexual functioning or to advanced stages of presbyrectia.

But this does not mean that every patient with a slightly abnormal NPT or some softening of his erections, or those with mild abnormalities in their penile circulation, should have injections or surgery. The organic deficits of older men are severe enough to preclude sexual functioning in only a minority of cases. The majority of our older patients, even those with minor physical problems, have retained sufficient sexual reserves so they ought to be able to function. However, they may become totally impotent because of their psychological problems and these patients are good candidates for sex therapy. For these reasons, in addition to evaluating the patient's physical deficits, it is also important to assess his remaining sexual capacities in order to determine if a trial of psychological treatment makes sense as a first-line treatment.

It should be remembered that intracavernosal injections of vasoactive substances, while essentially safe, are not entirely benign. A few patients find the injections painful and some develop bruises and nodules on their penis. In addition, systemic complications have been reported, although they are extremely rare (see Chapter III). If there are no other treatment options, these small risks are certainly worth taking. However, if he has sufficient remaining erectile capacity, it is often to the patient's best interest to attempt to restore his sexual functioning with psychological therapies prior to considering physical means such as ICI.

SEX THERAPY WITH OLDER PATIENTS

If the physical evaluation reveals that the patient has sufficient erectile reserve, and if he has a cooperative partner, a trial of sex therapy is indicated. Sex therapy is often successful with older patients, especially when they have had a history of good sexual functioning prior to the onset of their age-related difficulties.

The aims of sex therapy with older patients and couples are to improve their sexual techniques and to reduce their sexual anxieties. The first step consists of reconceptualizing their problem realistically and helping them to accept their limitations. At the same time, it is important to maintain a positive, optimistic attitude about their remaining capacities. I always sit down with the patient (or the couple, if he has a partner) and discuss the physical findings, stressing his remaining sexual reserves as well as the limitations. I might show the couple the NPT record and tell the patient, "You do have some softening of your erections and it looks like it will be difficult for you to have an erection in the evenings. But look here. In the morning you have pretty good erections. In other words, as you suspected, you have developed some physical problems. But these are only mild. Your sexual difficulty has become more serious than it should be because of your emotional reactions. I think you could learn to function again if you are willing to modify your sexual techniques."

The Therapeutic Exercises

The therapeutically structured sexual interactions that are used in sex therapy for patients with psychogenic impotence will be described in Chapter VIII. These "sexual homework assignments" are excellent for treating younger men with psychogenic erectile difficulties. In addition, if they are modified to compensate for the older couple's special emotional and physical limitations and to maximize their remaining capacities, they are very effective with this patient population also. Following are some examples of therapeutic behavioral assignments that we have found useful with patients over 50.

Often, the first therapeutic assignment for men with

psychogenic impotence is the Sensate Focus I (SF-I) exercise. During this phase of treatment, intercourse is prohibited while the couple take turns gently caressing each other's bodies. These nondemanding sensuous experiences are excellent for reducing performance anxiety because this exposure often produces spontaneous erections in younger men without any direct genital stimulation. However, many normal older men lose their capacity for attaining spontaneous erections and they may not become hard from exchanging body caresses with the partner even if this is subjectively arousing. Because this could upset the couple and reinforce the patient's sense of failure and his negative anticipations, we usually skip Sensate Focus I with older men and start the assignments with the Sensate Focus II exercises.

During this assignment, the couple also refrain from intercourse and orgasm. The partners begin sexual contact by caressing each other's bodies sensuously as in SF-I. In addition, when they feel aroused they then take turns stimulating each other's genitalia gently and slowly. Such nondemanding physical stimulation of the penis frequently provokes erections in older men, even if they have lost the capacity to erect spontaneously in response to psychic stimulation alone, and this can be very encouraging.

The next behavioral step with older patients may be the exchange of orgasm, without intercourse (SF-III). In this therapeutic exercise, the couple is asked to use lubricants and to take turn stimulating each other's genitalia manually to orgasm. One of the purposes of this assignment is to broaden beyond coitus the older patient's conception of what constitutes normal or successful sex. This is important because the combination of the softer erections and dryer vaginas of the elderly makes penetration increasingly difficult.

In certain cases, we ask the patient to close his eyes and focus on his favorite erotic fantasy while his partner stimulates him or, if this is not offensive to either partner, while watching erotic videotapes. This allows the man to "tune out" his performance anxiety, which becomes increasingly difficult to tolerate as he ages.

When this is compatible with the couple's value system, we might suggest that they experiment with oral sex, which can be very helpful for enhancing the erections of older men; it is also very pleasing to many women. This often necessitates that the therapist work through a partner's long-standing guilt, shame, and aversion for this form of stimulation during the therapy sessions.

The Therapy Sessions

In addition to educating the patient about the effects of aging and introducing more effective sexual techniques, in most cases the therapist must also deal with emotional issues. When they are young and sexually vigorous, men can often function despite the remnants of the antisexual conditioning of their childhood, despite some degree of sexual insecurity, despite the existence of some unresolved intrapsychic conflict, and despite the presence of a certain amount of latent marital hostility. However, as people age and as their sexuality becomes more fragile, all of these old problems tend to resurface and create potency difficulties, as well as resistances to treatment.

The following are some of the deeper issues that commonly come up in sex therapy with elderly patients.

Men's increasing sexual dependence on women. The assignments that are prescribed for older couples often entail the wife's taking a more active role in lovemaking, while the husband learns to accept a more passive or more receiving position. Not surprisingly, such unfamiliar and previously avoided experiences and role shifts can be upsetting to either or both partners. The older man's greater dependence on his partner can rekindle long-buried feelings of ambivalence towards women in men who have never completely gotten over their problems with their mothers. Sometimes, when such men find themselves once again in a dependent position, they displace the rage that they once felt towards their rejecting or over-controlling mothers onto their current partner. Not surprisingly, the husband's unwarranted hostility does not inspire their wives' enthusiastic cooperation in bed.

Erotica and fantasy. Although patients frequently relish the doctor's "permission" to enjoy erotica and sexual fantasies, this can also create problems. Rejection-sensitive wives are often threatened by the therapist's suggestion that their husband attempt to "tune out" their performance anxieties and obsessions by focusing on these sexual fantasies. If the woman is emotionally fragile, she may misinterpret her partner's arousal by the image of another woman as a devastating, personal rejection. There are several cases in our files where a poor therapeutic outcome could be directly attributed to our inability to resolve the wife's resistance to erotica and our failure to get her to see that her aging husband's desire for fantasy was not a personal insult to her, but rather his attempt to avoid disappointing her by losing his erection.

The therapist's suggestion that a couple try erotic videotapes or books or his encouragement that the patient focus on his fantasies during lovemaking can also mobilize resistances in conventional individuals, whose religious or traditional background has conditioned them to feel guilty and ashamed about their sexual feelings and fantasies, especially if these vary from the norm.

Such inhibitions must be worked through before patients can fully embrace the therapist's "permission" to enjoy their sexuality and to engage in previously taboo sexual behavior. A strong, positive therapeutic alliance with the therapist and an identification with his or her more liberal sexual values is the key to the resolution of such "cultural" obstacles to the sexual rehabilitation of the older patient.

Marital hostilities. Not infrequently, the age-related sexual changes create an emotional crisis that can evoke latent marital hostilities and resistances to treatment. The therapist's inability to resolve the couple's anger is the greatest single cause of treatment failure in sex therapy of older couples.

In one common scenario, the aging man's growing sexual dependency gives his wife, who may have felt helplessly angry, and at the mercy of her controlling, aggressive, difficult husband throughout the early years of their marriage, the perfect opportunity to get even. Such passive-aggressive wives do not usually refuse the sexual requests of their husbands directly. Instead, they act out their anger in various and subtle ways. Some succeed in "castrating" their husbands simply by withholding their acceptance and support, which become increasingly critical to maintaining sexual functioning as a man ages. Others express their anger by their passivity and unresponsiveness in bed. Still others manage to undermine their partner's sexual confidence with criticisms of his sexual functioning or by making inappropriate performance demands. The wife's claims that, "I am not a morning person, I feel romantic only at night," when she knows full well that he now has trouble functioning at night, is a common, seemingly innocent expression of sexual sabotage.

It is equally common for an angry husband to punish his wife for his own sexual decline by becoming neglectful or by rejecting her. We often see men who have been engaged in long-standing marital power struggles withdraw from their wives emotionally and avoid sex when their own potency becomes more fragile. These passive-aggressive men do not openly communicate their sexual needs and vulnerabilities to their wives. Instead, they create the impression that their impotence is *her* fault, implying that if she were younger and more attractive there would be no problem. Such a cruel pattern of detachment and blame can last for years, leaving the vulnerable post-menopausal wife feeling rejected and devastated and hardly in the mood to be a cooperative partner.

Many older couples who seek help to restore their sexual functioning have been too angry at each other for too long to be able to commit themselves to or to benefit from a treatment that aims at increasing their intimacy and their pleasure together. Such adversarial couples require prior conjoint counseling in order to resolve their marital conflicts before it makes sense to deal with the husband's impotence with sex therapy and/or with pharmacological treatment.

THE ROLE OF INJECTION THERAPY IN THE TREATMENT OF OLDER IMPOTENT MEN

Intracavernosal injections are an ideal treatment for older men who are not good candidates for psychological treatment. They are also an excellent alternative to penile implant surgery, which requires general anesthesia and entails the long-term placement of foreign material inside the patient's body, especially now that the question of the safety of silicone implants has been raised.

Sex therapy is not the answer for every older patient with sexual complaints. For one, expert sex therapy is not yet available in every country and in every community; in such circumstances injection therapy is a reasonable therapeutic alternative.

Also, some older patients are not amenable to sex therapy because they are too set in their ways. Again, in our experience many older couples in our culture have a gratifying response to sex therapy. Thus, it is not unusual for a couple to report that they feel sexually liberated by their experience in therapy and are so much closer to each other emotionally that they are now having the best sex of their lives. But other older persons are simply too rigid to be able to change their sexual behavior and techniques in ways that would help them adapt.

A couple may have been accustomed to a certain sexual routine that has worked for them since the beginning of their relationship. They have sex only in evenings, with a minimum of foreplay, in the male superior position, with little genital stimulation and with no communication. After 30, 40, or even 50 years of this routine, some older persons are understandably reluctant to begin experimenting with oral sex or erotica or to have sex in the morning (when the older man's erections are stronger). At the age of 60, 70, or even 80, it is difficult for some women who have played a passive sexual role all their lives to suddenly start taking responsibility for their husband's erections, and to learn to stimulate his genitalia actively and for as long as it takes to get him to function. And it is equally difficult for some men who have never been open with their wives to begin to make themselves vulnerable by expressing their innermost fears and desires. For such inflexible couples, injection therapy can be an excellent alternative that can enable them to resume sexual relations without the necessity of changing their behavior.

The following case is typical.

CASE 8.—INJECTION THERAPY FOR AN INFLEXIBLE OLDER COUPLE

The husband, H, was an 80-year-old retired successful real estate developer. He was a tall, energetic, and healthy man whose interest in sex had not diminished with age. But Mrs. H, a petite pretty woman age 75, his wife of 55 years, was resisting his overtures and avoiding sex as much as she could without causing a fight. This was out of character for this couple. Mrs. H was an agreeable woman who liked to make her husband happy and they had always enjoyed a harmonious relationship. In the past, before the onset of his age-related changes, her mere physical presence had been sufficient to arouse him and the couple had a satisfactory sex life together for many years.

Now, with the onset of his presbyrectia, Mr. H needed her to be much more active and to provide him with lengthier physical stimulation of his genitalia in order to attain and maintain his erections. He had no hesitation about demanding this from her, nor about asking her to watch erotic videotapes with him. She did not like to refuse him, but she felt very uncomfortable with these new sexual demands, which were contrary to her ladylike habits and traditional values. She hated to be awakened early to take advantage of his morning erections before she had a chance to brush her teeth and comb her hair, and although she overcame her reluctance about oral sex, she grew tired of fellating him if this took more than a minute. Also, his obsessive pressuring for sex was getting to her and she was developing a sexual aversion.

H had been told by his urologist that there was nothing physically wrong with him. But this was not really true. While the patient did not have a specific disease state, such as diabetes or a hormone deficiency, there was a significant age-related softening and fragility to his erections; this was not detected by the doctor.

Since he had been told that he was "OK," he blamed his wife and her "sexual problems" for his impotence. However, she was unable to summon more enthusiasm for lovemaking, and he felt so hurt and angry at her for "rejecting" him that he threatened to find a young mistress. At this juncture, the couple consulted me to find out if sex therapy could help Mrs. H to become "more interested" in sex.

There was really nothing wrong with Mrs. H's sexual response (she was on replacement therapy and still lubricating and having orgasms). The problem was Mr. H's erections, which had become deficient. But

Mrs. H had absolutely no interest in exploring new sexual techniques that might help him function. However, she had no objections to the intercavernosal injections.

H had an excellent response to VIP and Phentolamine and the couple were able to resume their mutually satisfying sexual relationship without having to change their sexual behavior pattern. Both were delighted with the results, although it took some effort to persuade H to limit his use of the injections to twice a week.

Single Older Men

Many older men who find themselves single after years of marriage are impotent when they try to have sex with new partners, although in the past they had had no sexual problems. Many of these men feel so humiliated by their anticipation of a sexual failure that, although they are lonely and starved for affection, they avoid socializing and don't seek the new relationships they so desperately need. Injection therapy can be a "lifesaver" for these patients.

The following case is typical.

CASE 9.—THE TEMPORARY USE OF INJECTIONS BY A WIDOWER

The patient, I, was an attractive, successful, 63-year-old widower. He had been happily married for 38 years to a woman who had died after a long, painful, terminal illness. The couple had married when they were in their early twenties and I's wife had been his first and only sexual partner. After a brief episode of "honeymoon impotence," the couple had had no sexual difficulties throughout their many years together. During her illness, he was extremely attentive to her. By mutual consent, they had avoided sexual contact after the recurrence of her cancer four and a half years prior to her death. The patient did not masturbate because of his religious background (Roman Catholic) and he had been completely celibate for the past six years.

One year after his wife's death, the patient began to date. The first time he tried to have sex, he lost his erection and, although the woman was supportive and encouraging, he was so ashamed that he never saw her again. The same thing happened with his two next partners.

Recently, the patient met a woman who really interested him and with whom he wanted a permanent relationship. Although he felt very attracted, he had not tried to make love to her because he feared that he would again be unable to perform. He was seeking help now, because he was afraid he would lose her if he continued to avoid sex.

The medical workup indicated some mild abnormalities. But the patient's sexual history revealed that he still had firm nocturnal and morning erections and this suggested that he had sufficient remaining erectile reserves to warrant a trial of sexual therapy.

Psychosexual therapy or counseling for single dysfunctional patients is based on the same integrated model as couple's sex therapy. More specifically, the patient is given therapeutic social and sexual "homework assignments."

These strategic interventions are backed up by office sessions with the therapist, which provide the opportunity to
explore the emotional issues that are often brought to the
surface by the patient's experiences.

With older single men, the thrust of counseling is on
education regarding the normal age-related changes in the
male sexual response, as well as on conveying realistic goals
and expectations. It may also be necessary, in the case of
recent widowers, to help them overcome their guilt about
being alive and enjoying sex again.

In addition, men who have not dated in many years may
avoid socializing and seeking sexual opportunities because
they are out of practice and have lost their confidence.
Such patients need help in improving their social and communication skills in order to overcome their avoidance.
And when they are ready to initiate sex with a new partner,
these men need strategies for making themselves comfortable in the sexual situation, and for protecting themselves
from their self-induced performance pressures. This
requires that the patient let down his defenses and that he
learn to communicate his sexual and emotional needs to
his new partner. In addition, men, just like women, have
to learn to say "no" to sexual invitations unless they feel
quite ready for this. In our "macho" culture, where "real"
men are expected to jump at any sexual opportunity, this
may prove difficult for the older man.

This process was pretty threatening for this traditional,
nonintimate man who had never been open about sex and
who had always related to women by pleasing and performing. He couldn't imagine "a gentleman" turning
down a woman's sexual invitation. It would have made him
feel vulnerable and exposed to ask a woman to accept less
than "perfect" functioning from him. In short, he was

reluctant to try to change his behavior at this point in his life.

But he was very interested in the injection program and he had an excellent response to papaverine.

The control that he now felt over his erections diminished his performance anxiety and obviated the need to change his approach to women. With the injections, he could still perform and please; this enabled him to risk proceeding with the relationship. He was able to perform "perfectly" with the injections, but he used these only a few times. His new partner proved to be a most accepting, loving, and sexually open woman who quickly put him at ease. After a few months of this "therapeutic" relationship, and with the therapist's support and encouragement, he became so comfortable with her that the injections became unnecessary.

Elderly men may experience some special problems with self-injection. Poor eyesight, obesity, and tremors can make injecting oneself into the penis difficult. Often, the wives will have to do the injecting. However, it is very much worth the physician's while to work patiently with his older patients to help them overcome these obstacles because the rewards can be great.

As a result of our increasing understanding of the pathogenesis of sexual dysfunctions in the elderly, and such recent advances in sexual medicine as the new injection treatment, the sexual functioning of many elderly patients can be restored or materially improved. The prognosis is especially good for those couples who had enjoyed good sexual relationships prior to the onset of the age-related changes in their sexual functioning.

Clinicians should become aware that sex may become

more, not less, important in a person's life with the passage
of time, because sexuality is a potentially enduring source
of pleasure and emotional well-being at a time when more
and more losses must be accepted and fewer and fewer
gratifications remain available. For these reasons, the restoration of sexual functioning can be a tremendous gift
to the older person and most gratifying for the physician.

CHAPTER VIII

Injection Therapy for Psychogenic Impotence

by Helen Singer Kaplan

THE ROLE OF intracavernosal injections in the treatment of psychogenic impotence is still controversial.

One group of physicians favor the use of pharmacotherapy, claiming good, long-term results in patients with psychogenic erectile dysfunctions (Lue & Tangano, 1987; Watters et al., 1988). Some of the urologists who recommend injection therapy for psychogenic impotence advise limiting this to patients who do not have access to sex therapy or to those who find psychological treatment is unacceptable (Dhabuwala et al., 1989). Others routinely administer intracavernosal injections of vasoactive substances to impotent patients regardless of etiology, as a first-line therapy, without offering psychological alternatives or adjuvant psychiatric support.

Some psychologically minded clinicians have a contrary view and consider the injection of vasoactive substances into the penises of men whose problems have a psychological basis as inappropriate and dangerous. There are psychoanalysts who have gone so far as to suggest that the use of pharmacological agents to provoke erections in men with physically normal genitalia smacks of "clockwork orange" and is medically un-ethical.

Our own position is in the center. We believe that injection therapy should *not* be used as a first-line treatment for men with psychogenic erectile dysfunction, nor should ICI be administered to such patients without proper psychiatric evaluation and support. Ethical considerations aside, this is not usually in the best interests of psychogenic patients because the benefits of injection treatment with this population tend to be very short-lived unless pharmacotherapy is administered within the context of sex therapy or psychotherapy (Althof et al., 1987; Turner et al., 1989). Moreover, there are risks of adversive psychiatric reactions when the injections are given to psychogenically impotent men without adequate psychiatric backup.

However, our clinical experience suggests that in certain cases of psychogenic erectile dysfunction the combined use of pharmacotherapy and sex therapy is warranted and potentially very useful. In fact, in some instances this combination is more effective than either modality by itself. More specifically, I have seen excellent results with the adjuvant use of intercavernosal injections in the following situations: 1. to "bypass" intractable performance anxiety when this creates an obstacle to the process of sex therapy; 2. in certain stalled sex therapy cases where injection therapy can be an effective addition to the armamentarium of methods we use to manage resistances to the behavioral modification of the patient's sexual symptom; and 3. for certain patients with psychogenic impotence who are not amenable to psychological treatment and for whom injection therapy offers an attractive alternative to celibacy or surgery.

PSYCHOGENIC IMPOTENCE

Anxiety is the "final common pathway" via which a variety of cultural, psychological, and relationship stressors converge to produce erectile failures in men with normal genitalia (Kaplan, 1974a). More specifically, it is the physiological (sympathetic) concomitant of sexual fear or anxiety that disrupts the erectile reflexes.

The physiology of penile erection has been described by Dr. Wagner in Chapter II. There it was explained that an erection is produced by a reversible high blood pressure system in the penis, which extends the organ and makes it rigid. When a man becomes sexually aroused, the penile arteries dilate. This increases the flow of blood into the penis. At the same time, the relaxation of certain smooth muscles within the corpora create a tamponade, which acts like a tourniquet to impede the outflow. By means of this mechanism, the blood is trapped at a high pressure within the fascia of the penis and this produces a rigid erection.

The physiological consequences of anxiety reverse this process. The experience of anxiety is not just a mental or cognitive CNS event. Fear or anxiety is automatically accompanied by a sympathetic surge that releases adrenaline and noradrenaline from the adrenal gland into the circulation. These "emergency" hormones reach the penis almost instantly, causing the penile arteries to constrict and the smooth muscles, which in their relaxed state held back the outflow, to constrict. This results in the rapid collapse of the erection.

The sympathetic surge that accompanies the feeling of anxiety is physically always the same and always equally incompatible with erection. The psychological origin or meaning of the patient's anxiety is entirely irrelevant to these mental processes. In other words, the body's physical response is identical whether or not the patient consciously recognizes that he is afraid. Moreover, it makes no difference if the source of the patient's anxiety is religious guilt about sexual pleasure, the unreasonable sexual demands of his hostile partner, or a long standing neurotic conflict about sex.

Performance Anxiety

In the great majority of cases, the immediate or final psychological trigger of the andrenergic surge that causes psychogenic impotence is *sexual performance anxiety*. A single episode of erectile failure in an inexperienced or insecure man can sometimes initiate a self-reinforcing cycle of failure and anticipation of failure, escalating into chronic and serious impotence. Such a vicious cycle of performance anxiety can occur in men who function well in other respects and are in good relationships; it is the sole cause of the problem for many patients who suffer from psychogenic impotence. In other cases, the patient's anxiety about performing sexually is only the "tip of the iceberg" and reflects his deeper sexual conflicts or relationship problems.

The Treatment of Psychogenic Impotence

The primary aim of all psychological treatments for psychogenic erectile disorders is to diminish the patient's performance anxiety. If this can be accomplished, the patient will be cured and regain his potency irrespective of any other psychological difficulties he may have. Conversely, if therapy does not succeed in diminishing the patient's performance anxiety and in making him comfortable in the sexual situation, his erectile dysfunction will not improve even if he attains valid insights into the deeper dynamics of his psychological difficulties through psycho-analysis and even if his relationship with his partner improves greatly with marital therapy.

Sex therapy is considered the treatment of choice for most patients with psychogenic impotence. This brief treatment method differs from other types of psychotherapy in that it focuses solely on improving the patient's sexual function-ing, and combines behavioral with psychodynamic tech-niques.

The behavioral aspect of treatment is composed of ther-apeutically structured sexual interactions that are designed to lower the patient's sexual anxiety in a gradual, systematic manner. The purpose of the exercises is to expose the patient to sexual situations that are pleasurable but not performance-oriented in order to sever the link between sex and performance anxiety. The following is a typical sequence of assignments that are carried out by the symptomatic patient and his partner in the privacy of their home.

1. The initial behavioral assignment for impotent patients is often the *Sensate Focus Exercise*, (SF-I) (see page 152). Again, during this exercise the couple refrain from inter-course; instead they alternately caress each other gently and slowly (Masters & Johnson, 1970). This intervention, which is designed to shift the patient's focus toward the mutual exchange of pleasure and away from performance concerns, is an excellent tactic for reducing performance

anxiety. Patients are frequently able to forget their obsessions about functioning and obtain spontaneous erections in response to these sensuous, nondemanding experiences, and this can begin to disrupt the cycle of the patient's performance anxiety impotence.

2. When the couple are comfortable with being nude together and touching each other, the next assignment often is *Sensate Focus II* (SF-II) (Kaplan, 1979, 1987). The essence of this exercise is that the partners continue to caress each other sensuously, but, in addition, they take turn stimulating each other's genitalia. During this phase of the program, the genitalia are stroked only in a teasing way, and not with the rhythmic tempo that leads to orgasm. This allows the exchange of pleasurable erotic sensations between the partners without the imposition of any performance requirements.

3. If the patient's anxiety has diminished to a point where he is now regularly having erections with his partner, we usually proceed to intravaginal containment in the *female superior position*. During this exercise, the patient lies on his back with his eyes closed, focusing his attention on his erotic sensation or on a sexual fantasy, while his partner stimulates his penis manually, using a lubricant. When he has a good erection, she guides his penis into her vagina while she is on top of him. Initially, the couple is instructed to interrupt coitus after a few thrusts, before the man ejaculates. After the patient has become accustomed to being erect inside his partner's vagina, the couple gradually proceed to intravaginal ejaculation.

This may sound like a "mechanical" treatment, but it is not. Although the behavioral protocol always follows this general model of an "in vivo" exposure to and desensitization of sexual anxiety, the program is modi-

fied to accommodate the needs of each patient and couple in a highly flexible manner. Thus, in actual practice,
few couples receive their assignments precisely as described above.

This program of systematic exposure to the pleasures
of sex devoid of performance pressure is highly effective
in restoring the potency of men with simple performance-
anxiety impotence. However, many patients and their partners have concomitant deeper problems and tend to resist
the rapid behavioral modification of their sexual symptom. They may also find the process of sex therapy, which
entails highly erotic and intimate experiences, quite
threatening.

The resolution of resistance is a major function of the
psychotherapeutic aspects of sex therapy. In the attempt to
keep treatment brief and symptom-focused, when we
encounter resistances we first try to "bypass" or "bridge
over" with behavioral and cognitive interventions the
patient's deeper conflicts that have caused therapeutic
impasse (Kaplan, 1974a, 1979, 1980, 1987).

Thus, if a couple has failed to do their sexual assignments correctly, or if they have manifested resistances in
some other manner, we will *repeat* and *modify the behavioral*
prescriptions so that these will evoke less anxiety. For
example, some rejection-sensitive patients panic during
Sensate Focus exercises because they are ashamed to let
their partners see them without an erection. In such a case,
I might suggest that they caress each other in the dark or
that the patient initially keep his underwear on. This couple would not proceed to caressing each other while nude,
with the lights on, until they are emotionally ready. At the
same time, during the therapy sessions we continue to support the couple's sexual growth and we keep on confront-

ing them with their sexual self-sabotage and with their resistances to treatment until these are resolved.

Such "strategic" tactics are often effective in overcoming a couple's resistance to improving their sexual functioning even in the presence of considerable psychopathology and/or marital disharmony. But if this fails and the patient's potency does not show rapid improvement, we then shift to a psychodynamic mode and attempt to foster insight into his deeper unconscious sexual conflicts. To this end, we explore childhood issues to greater depth, and make active use of dream material (Kaplan, 1979, 1980, 1983, 1987).

INTRACORPORAL INJECTION AS AN ADJUVANT TO SEX THERAPY

Within this theoretical framework, we are now using injection therapy with certain psychogenically impotent men who are having trouble cooperating with and responding to sex therapy. In some of these cases, the injections are used as a temporary adjuvant to psychological treatment and to "bypass" intractable performance anxiety. In other instances, the intracavernosal injections offer an ongoing solution for patients who fail to improve with psychological treatment.

The temporary use of pharmacologically induced erections can, in some cases, effectively "bypass" intractable performance anxiety, which is a major source of treatment failure in psychogenic impotence. More specifically, the knowledge that they can attain erections by injection can instill enough confidence in men who cannot overcome their performance anxiety and their sexual avoidance so that they can risk engaging in the therapeutic, structured, sexual interactions with their partners. For similar reasons, the adjuvant use of injection therapy can be especially helpful with single, impotent patients who are avoiding socializing and finding partners because of their anticipatory fears of sexual failure.

The Single Patient

Although sex therapy was originally designed for use with couples only, the strategy of combining therapeutically structured sexual interactions with psychodynamically oriented psychotherapy can be successfully adapted for treating single patients with psychosexual dysfunctions (also see Chapter VII).

This is a very important development in this age of AIDS, which has made the use of surrogate partners very risky (for the patient as well as for the surrogate), and the advice to patients that they find casual sexual partners to "practice" with, unconscionable.

Injection therapy has a definite place in the treatment of single, impotent men who are caught in the "Catch 22" dilemma of avoiding sexual encounters that could help them get over their performance anxieties because they are afraid that they will not be able to perform with a new partner. The following case vignette illustrates the value of combining psychotherapy and pharmacotherapy to treat a single impotent man with intractable performance anxiety.

CASE **10.** **THE TEMPORARY USE OF INJECTIONS TO BYPASS**
INTRACTABLE PERFORMANCE ANXIETY
IN A SINGLE MAN

The patient was an attractive, successful, divorced 44-year-old photographer who had a lifelong history of severe and recurrent performance anxiety impotence. J's sexual functioning had improved temporarily during his marriage, but he could function with his wife only if she said to him, "don't worry, you're going to be fine," prior to each and every sexual encounter. Time and repeated successful intercourse did nothing to extinguish this patient's obsessive performance anxiety.

J had been impotent with two women after his divorce five years ago. A highly perfectionistic, compulsive, achievement-oriented man, he was so distressed and humiliated by his failure that he avoided dating and became reclusive, devoting himself compulsively to his photographic work at which he excelled. But his loneliness and his lack of pleasure in life caused him to feel increasingly depressed.

This patient had truly intractable, obsessive performance anxiety that had survived marital therapy, psychoanalysis, and pharmacotherapy. He had undergone couple therapy when his marriage broke up, followed by long-term psychodynamically oriented psychotherapy. In addition, he had a course of anti-panic medication (imipramine [Tofrani] and alprezolam [xanax]) for his panic attacks and phobia about flying.

Through his work in therapy, he gained valid insights into the childhood origins of his vulnerabilities, his phobias, and his overreaction to rejection by women. He also proved to be an excellent responder to tricyclic medication and Xanax (aprezolam). His panic attacks abated and he was soon able to fly without any difficulty. In response to these treatments, this patient became completely functional in every other respect, but his severe sexual performance anxiety did not show any improvement. He continued to avoid socializing and his sense of isolation deepened.

In a final attempt to bypass this patient's intractable performance anxiety, I offered him the option of pharmacotherapy. J was most eager to try this and, since his genitalia were normal, he achieved excellent erections with ICI.

The patient "practiced" injecting himself and masturbating to erotic videos while he was alone. He was pleased when this worked "perfectly" for five consecutive trial runs, giving this perfectionistic man the courage to begin to go out with women again.

The first time he was going to go to bed with a woman, he had every intention of using the injection. He left the carefully prepared paraphernalia in the bathroom and reassured himself with the thought, "it will work perfectly with the injection."

However, he became so excited and firm that he didn't need the injections and had successful intercourse without the interference of his old nemesis, his performance anxiety. J felt elated and began to date again.

Now that J was no longer hiding behind his potency problem, we had the opportunity in the therapy sessions to analyze in greater depth his long-standing painful overreaction to criticism or rejection from his sexual partners. These sources of upset had their origin in his problems with his mother, which he had never fully resolved before. A totally narcissistic woman, who could still make him fly into a rage, she had paid little attention to him as a boy and always compared him unfavorably with a gifted cousin. In the attempt to gain his mother's approval, J had developed a compulsive need to perform "perfectly," first in school and later at work.

This patient is now off all medications. For the past eight months, he has been living with an attractive, sexy woman. During this time, he has had to use the injections only twice. The idea that this "fail safe" is always available if he should need it has been so reassuring to him that he almost never needs to make use of it. J now has an active sex life with a new lover and is enjoying his life. Again, he hardly ever uses the injections, but he has made a habit out of checking that all is in order before he makes love. And, with my encouragement, he renews his supply every three months.

The rapid improvement of a patient's potency by means of the intracavernosal injections can be gratifying, as it was in the case cited above. But this can be potentially hazardous when the symptom of sexual inadequacy has served as a defense against the emergence of deeper pathology. However, in the hands of a skilled psychotherapist, the elimination of the defense of impotence can also create a therapeutic opportunity.

When used within a psychodynamic framework, which exploits the exposure of the patient's underlying conflicts that can be brought about by the removal of his sexual symptom, the combined use of sex therapy and pharmacotherapy produces benefits that can sometimes extend beyond the restoration of potency, to facilitating insights into the patient's deeper problems. In fortunate cases, this can lead to lasting improvement in a couple's relationship. Once the question of attaining and maintaining an erection has been "bypassed" by the injections and is no longer an emotional issue, the patient and his partner are then confronted with and have the opportunity to resolve their deeper sexual fears and marital problems during the conjoint therapy sessions. The following case vignette illustrates how the temporary use of injection therapy stripped away a patient's psychological defenses and lured his underlying neurotic problems with women to the surface of his consciousness, making these accessible to the therapeutic process.

CASE 11. PSYCHOGENIC IMPOTENCE AS A NEUROTIC DEFENSE*

The patient, K, was a 55-year-old, hard-driving, highly successful, competitive businessman who for the past two months had been unable to maintain his erection with his new second wife, a beautiful model 25 years his junior.

The couple were in a crisis. They had been fighting constantly and bitterly and she had recently threatened to leave him. The thought of being abandoned by his new wife and the public humiliation he would have to endure utterly panicked this man. He was desperate to cure his impotence because he was convinced that this was the cause of his marital problems.

---

*This case was cited in a previous publication (Kaplan, 1989b).

Organic causes had been ruled out by the patient's competent urologist who referred him to us for sex therapy. But this sexually insecure, anxious, performance-oriented man objected to the Sensate Focus exercises. He simply couldn't tolerate the idea of abstaining from intercourse and "only" exchanging gentle, sensuous caresses with his wife, even for a little while. He feared that this would make him appear even more inadequate and "impotent" to her and would "turn her off" completely. The other alternative, long-term psychotherapy, was equally unpalatable to him.

I joined his resistance to admitting to himself that it was his aggressive personality, and not his impotence, that was upsetting his wife. I did this by suggesting that we might try pharmacotherapy combined with psychological counseling. The idea that he would have physical control over his erections appealed to K greatly, he was able to obtain excellent erections by injecting himself with prostaglandin E_1 and phentolamine. This enabled the couple to have lengthy, physically satisfying intercourse on several occasions.

However, there was no parallel improvement in this couple's relationship. In fact, their fights and power struggles became more frequent and increasingly bitter.

Now that the potency issue was moot, K had to face his deeper emotional problems and his underlying difficulties with women. He came to realize that he could function perfectly well without any physical aids when he was getting along well with his wife and when he felt loved and appreciated by her. When it became clear to him that he was impotent only when she was angry with him or cold, he discontinued the injections.

At the same time in his therapy sessions, this patient began to see that it was the mounting rage he felt towards his wife and his attempts to control and bully her, not his potency problem, that were poisoning the relationship. His fury towards his wife was a replay of the anger he once felt at his mother, a critical, controlling, demanding woman whom he had never been able to please despite his considerable efforts and achievements. The symptom of impotence had served as a defense against the emergence of these painful childhood memories. Once this symptom was removed by the injections, K had to face these issues in his therapy sessions.

K began to realize that he was continually provoking his wife to anger. He also saw that his choosing her had a neurotic basis. In marrying this distant, narcissistic, and perfectionistic woman who was like his mother in many respects, he had denied his deep need for emotional closeness to and approval from a woman. But he had been obsessed by her beauty, which made him feel like a "winner" again after his painful divorce.

This couple eventually separated. But K had gained sufficient insight into the origins of his problems with women so that he stopped sabotaging his sexuality by trying to function with hostile, rejecting partners. He found that he was potent with more supportive lovers without the use of injections.

On follow-up a year later, he was having a harmonious, romantic relationship with a much more suitable partner. This woman was not a great beauty nor a "trophy." More important, she was extremely accepting and loving, enabling him to relate to her without his old provocativeness and anger.

Deeper Causes of Resistance

The deeper psychological causes of potency problems and resistances to treatment often involve the patient's unresolved negative feelings for his mother, which he transfers to his sexual partner as an adult. The malignant influence of early problems with the mother were illustrated in the case vignettes of J, the anxious photographer, and K, the remarried businessman. Both men had mothers for whom they could never perform well enough, and who were cruel to them in their self-involvement. When they grew up, they then had the same expectations of their partners, namely that the women would be demanding and rejecting, and this fueled their sexual anxieties.

But painful childhood interactions with a harsh, intimidating, or emotionally distant father can also predispose a man to excessive sexual anxiety and sexual dysfunction. We have seen many cases of men who could not overcome their potency problems or their resistance to treatment until they had gained insight into and resolved their painful relationships with their competitive fathers.

In addition to these intrapsychic conflicts, which originate in the vicissitudes of the child's early experiences with his family, culturally determined negative attitudes about sex also play a significant role in the deeper psychic infrastructure of the sexual problems of many patients. It is difficult for a man to abandon himself to his sexual pleasures if he has been "programmed" when he was in his formative years to regard sex as dirty, dangerous, sinful, and something you would never ask a nice woman to do.

The doctor's caring attitude and encouragement of the patient's sexuality, the very act of his or her offering to help the patient become potent, can go a long way towards ameliorating such deeper obstacles to sexual health. However, the therapist's "permission" is not sufficient in every case, and some patients need to attain insight before they can free their sexuality from the shackles of their pasts.

INTRACORPORAL INJECTIONS IN INTRACTABLE PSYCHOGENIC IMPOTENCE

The following case vignette will illustrate the successful long-term use of the intracorporal injection for a patient with recurrent erectile failure who did not respond to psychological treatment.

CASE 12. SUCCESS WITH INJECTIONS AFTER SEX THERAPY FAILURE*

Mr. L was 62 and his wife 61. The couple had been married for 34 years and had raised two children. The husband had suffered from recurrent episodes of erectile dysfunction throughout the early years of their marriage. These were self-limiting and usually lasted three to four weeks. When he reached his fifties, however, he became chronically impotent and the couple sought sex therapy.

Mrs. L had been an attractive woman when she was

*This case was cited in a previous publication (Kaplan, 1989b).

young, but had become obese in her fifties and in recent years had developed some disabling medical problems.

L had been instantly attracted to his wife when they met 35 years ago and neither the physical changes she had undergone nor the deterioration of her health had diminished his ardor. The idea of masturbating or seeking another partner did not enter his mind and he continually pressured her for sex. Most of the time she rejected him, but once in a while she acquiesced, as long as it did not require "too much effort" or activity on her part.

We had seen Mr. and Mrs. L in our practice for sex therapy on and off for over eight years. They had an ambivalent relationship, which caused obstacles to successful sex therapy. The husband was an anxious, obsessive-compulsive man who was very dependent on his wife's approval. His excessive concerns about pleasing her, together with her negative attitude, intensified his sexual performance anxiety. The wife was a critical, self-absorbed woman. She was thoroughly disgusted with her husband's passivity and his anxieties. She was so angry that, although she understood that he needed this in order to function, she had resisted our encouragement, in the sex therapy sessions, to be more supportive to her husband and a more active sexual partner.

The couple had gained a good deal of insight into their problems with each other during the therapy, and each time Mr. L had responded with a temporary improvement of his sexual functioning. But this never lasted for more than a few months. He would then relapse into another cycle of obsessive performance-anxiety impotence, she would become enraged at him, and they would return for further therapy.

Last year, L called the office to complain that he was once again experiencing erectile difficulties. This time we offered him injection therapy. At first, he was afraid to inject himself and he obsessed about possible harmful effects. But he finally decided to try and was pleased to find that he was able to attain excellent erections.

Mrs. L was delighted to be absolved from responsibility for her husband's erections and for his anxiety. She had always preferred a passive-receptive role in bed and she longed for leisurely, relaxed intercourse. The injections have made this possible and the couple now have intercourse in a regular basis. Although he has no physical problems, they invariably use the injections when they make love.

CAUTIONS AND LIMITATIONS

In citing these successful cases, I do not wish to imply that the use of intracavernosal injections will make it possible to restore the potency of every patient with resistant psychogenic impotence. On the contrary, I believe that adjunctive pharmacotherapy is useful only in a small proportion of carefully selected patients with psychogenic erectile dysfunctions and that this treatment is most likely to be effective when this is used within the context of psychodynamically oriented sex therapy. Moreover, I have seen adversive psychiatric reactions when the injections are used with fragile patients by a clinician who does not understand the emotional meaning of the sexual symptom or of the ICI procedure for the patient and his partner.

According to psychoanalytic theory, the symptom of (psychogenic) impotence invariably serves as a defense against the emergence of deeper, unconscious sexual conflicts. The rapid removal of this symptom by means of behavior modification or intracavernosal injections exposes the patient to the dangers of a psychic catastrophe or to the development of substitute psychosomatic or psychological symptoms. This is the major basis for the objections of some psychoanalysts to the use of injection treatment with psychogenic erection problems.

However, our experience with over 5,000 patients with sexual disorders over the past 25 years indicates that this is not true, in the majority of cases. Most patients with psychosexual dysfunctions, like H, the obsessive man, I, the shy widower, and L, whose wife did not want to become more active, do not become depressed nor do they develop substitute symptoms when their potency improves rapidly in response to behavioral or pharmacological treatment. Actually, in our experience, in contrast to the many organically impotent patients who are jubilant with the results of ICI, most patients with psychogenic erectile dysfunctions show little psychological change, either for better or worse, after the rapid improvement of their sexual functioning. However, there are some, like J, the "perfectionist" in the last case study, who actually feel a lot better.*

Injection therapy was successful for K and for Mr. and Mrs. L because it was not administered before the therapist

---

*According to behavioral theory, the successful mastery of a symptom such as impotence is predicted to have a positive "ripple effect" on the patient's general psychological welfare. We have seen this, but in a relatively small number of patients.

had an in-depth understanding of the psychic infrastructure of these patients' sexual symptoms, and of the dynamics of their marital relationship. We knew beforehand that the injections would fit these patients' emotional needs and would not stir up latent hostilities nor remove any of their psychological defenses.

More specifically, we understood that neither K nor L was seriously ambivalent about making love to his wife, on any psychic level, and that it was only their persistent performance anxiety that stood in the way of their potency. Not surprisingly, when the injections "bypassed" their performance anxiety, they both functioned without difficulties. In fact, L actually experienced a positive ripple effect in that his depression lifted and his whole life seemed to go better.

Moreover, we also were careful not to suggest the use of injections to the Ls, until it was quite clear that this would not threaten Mrs. L. On the contrary, we knew that the injections would enable her to gratify her long-standing desire for hassle-free, lengthy sexual intercourse and we anticipated, correctly, that she would be entirely cooperative.

However, in some cases, fortunately a minority, the symptom of psychogenic impotence does seem to protect the patient from the emergence of underlying psychic pain. The rapid improvement of potency that is brought about by the injections poses a definite psychological hazard for these more fragile patients. For the same reasons, the injections are also psychologically dangerous for the partner if she has serious emotional problems. Thus, injection therapy for psychogenic impotence should be used with caution and reserved for patients who are free of serious, concomitant psychiatric problems.

As an example of the inappropriate use of injection therapy, I saw a 30-year-old man with an obsessive-compulsive personality disorder. This patient experienced a massive anxiety attack after he obtained an excellent erection in the urologist's office in response to an injection of Papaverine. This disturbed man's impotence had served as a defense against intolerable, unresolved oedipal issues, which threatened to emerge when he saw his erection and realized that he no longer had an excuse to avoid intercourse with his partner. He panicked and developed the obsession that the injection had done irreversible damage to his penile circulation. He then instituted a malpractice suit against the doctor.

As another example, I have seen a treatment failure which resulted in depression in the partner of a man with inhibited sexual desire due to a deep-seated intimacy-passion split. This patient was given injection therapy by his urologist and attained good erections, but he avoided using them. The mechanical tumescence provided by the vasoactive drug simply did not help him overcome his fears of melding erotic passion with emotional closeness; he could not bring himself to make love to his wife. Not surprisingly, his continued avoidance of sex in the face of his perfectly good erections took away all excuses and intensified the wife's feelings of frustration and despair.

I have observed an adversive reaction in a son of holocaust survivors. This man was so profoundly ambivalent about bringing children into a world that had destroyed his family that he was not amenable to psychoanalysis, sex therapy, or pharmacotherapy. After he received his injection material to take home, his girlfriend expected him to make love to her and he did so. However, he then broke down with a serious depression. This was precipitated by the mechanical removal of his impotence, which had served as a defense against his profound, unresolved, underlying pain.

In a similar vein, Turner and her colleagues (Althof et al., 1987) cite the case of a homosexual man who became depressed after he used the injection-induced erections to have intercourse with his wife. The attempt to override with ICI this man's desire to have sex with men is a good example of a highly inappropriate and manipulative misuse of this excellent treatment modality.

References

Adaikan, P.G. (1979). *Pharmacology of the human penis.* Ph.D. Thesis, University of Singapore, Singapore.

Alter, G.J., Rose, H.B., Tabencki, S., Podell, R.M. (1988). Comparison of penile systolic pressures and duplex sonography in assessment of arteriogenic impotence [abstract]. Boston: *Proceedings of the 3rd Biennial World Congress on Impotence, 29.*

Althof, S.E., Bodner, D. R., Turner, L. A., Levine, S. B., Risen, C. B., Kursh, E.D., & Resnick, M. I., (Fall, 1987). Intracavernosal injection in the treatment of impotence: A prospective study of sexual, psychological and marital functioning. *Journal of Sex & Marital Therapy, 13,* (3).

American Psychiatric Association (1980). *Diagnostic and Statistical Manual of Mental Disorders, Third Edition (DSM-III).* Washington, D.C.: American Psychiatric Association.

American Psychiatric Association (1992). *DSM-IV Option Book.* Washington, D.C.: American Psychiatric Association.

Andersson, K-E., Holmquist, F., & Wagner, G. (1991). Pharmacology of drugs used for treatment of erectile dysfunction and priapism. *International Journal of Impotence Research, 3,* 155–172.

Bondil, P., Louis, J. F., Daures, J. P., Costa, P., Lopez, C., Navratil, H. (1990). Clinical measurement of penile extensibility: Preliminary results. *International Journal of Impotence Research, 2,* 193–201.

Brecher, E. M., & the Editors of Consumer Reports Books (1984). *Love, Sex and Aging.* Boston: Little, Brown & Co.

Brindley, G. S. (1983a). Cavernosal alpha-blockade and human penile erection. *Journal of Physiology, 342,* 24P.

Brindley, G. S. (1983b). Cavernosal Alpha-Blockade: A new technique for investigating and treating erectile impotence. *British Journal of Psychiatry, 143,* 332–337.

Brindley, G. S., & Craggs, M. D. (1975). *Journal of Physiology, 256,* 55P.

Buvat, J., Buvat-Herbaut, M., Lemaire, A., & Marcolin, G. (1988). Les causes organiques cachées de l'impuissance. Methodes diagnostiques et évaluation critique de leur responsabilité. *Annales d'Urologie, 22,* 36–47.

Buvat, J., Buvat-Herbault, M., Lemaire, A., Marcolin, G., & Quittelier, E. (1990). Recent developments in the clinical assessment and diagnosis of erectile dysfunction. *Annual Review of Sex Research, 1,* 265–308.

Buvat, J., Lemaire, A., Buvat-Herbaut, M., & Marcolin, G. (1989). Safety of intracavernous injections using an alpha-blocking agent. *Journal of Urology, 141,* 1364–1367.

Buvat, J., Lemaire, A., Marcolin, G., Buvat-Herbaut, M., & Dehaene, J.L. (1989). Impuissance par fuite veineuse: á la recherche de críteres diagnostiques fiables [abstract]. *Proceedings of the 7th congress of the Société d' Andrologie de Langue Francaise, 27.*

Christ, G. J., Maayani, S., Valcic, M., & Melman, A. (1990). Pharmacological studies of human erectile tissue: characteristics of spontaneous contractions and alterations in α a-adrenoceptor responsiveness with age and disease in isolated tissue. *British Journal of Pharmacology; 101,* 375–381.

Crenshaw, T. L., & Goldberg, J. P. (In Press): *Sexual Pharmacology: Drugs That Affect Sexual Functioning.*

Crenshaw, T. L., Goldberg, J. P., & Stern, P. C. (Winter, 1987). Pharmacologic modification of sexual dysfunction. *Journal of Sex & Marital therapy, 13* (14).

De Groat, W. C., & Steers, W. D. (1988). Neuroanatomy and Neurophysiology of penile erection. In E. Tanagho et al. (Ed.), *Compentorary Management of Impotence and Infertility* (pp. 3–27). Baltimore: William & Wilkins.

DePalma, R. G., Edwards, C. M., Schwab, F. J., & Steinberg, D. L. (1988). Modern management of impotence associated with aortic surgery. In J. J. Bergan, J. S. T. Yao (Eds.), *Arterial Surgery: New Diagnostic and Operative Techniques* (pp. 328–337). Orlando: Grune & Stratton.

Dhabuwala, C. B., Kerkar, A., Bhutwala, A., & Pierce, J. M. (1990). Intracavernous papaverine in the management of psychogenic impotence. *Archives of Andrology, 24.*

Domer, F. R., Wessler, G., Brown, R. L., & Charles, H. C. (1978). Involvement of the sympathetic nervous system in the urinary bladder internal sphincter and in penile erection in the anesthetized cat. *Investigative Urology, 15,* 404–407.

Earle, C. M., Cherry, D. J., & Keogh, E. J. (1991). Interaction of amantidine and prostaglandin E_1. *International Journal of Impotence Research, 3,* 32.

Ebbehøj, J. (1975). A new operation for priapism. *Scandinavian Journal of Plastic and Reconstructive Surgery, 8,* 241–242.

Ebbehøj, J., Uhrenholt, A., & Wagner, G. (1980). Infusion cavernosography in the human in the unstimulated and stimulated situations and its diagnostic value. In A. W. Zorgniotti & G. Rossi (Eds.), Vasculogenic impotence: *Proceedings of 1st International Conference on Corpus Cavernosum Revascularization* (pp. 191–196). Springfield, IL: Charles C Thomas.

Ebbehøj, J., & Wagner, G. (1979). Insufficient penile erection due to abnormal drainage of cavernous bodies. *Urology, 13,* 507–510.

Forsberg, L., Gusta VII, B., Höjerback, T., & Olsson, A. M. (1979). Impotence, smoking and β-blocking drugs. *Fertility and Sterility, 31,* 589–591.

Freud, S. (1961). *The Complete Works of Sigmund Freud* (pp. 213–222). London: Hogarth.

Fuchs, A. M., Mehringer, C. M., & Rajfer, J. (1989). Anatomy of penile venous drainage in potent and impotent men during cavernosography. *Journal of Urology, 141,* 1353–1356.

George, L.K., & Weiler, S. J. (1981). Sexuality in middle and late life. *Archives of General Psychiatry, 38.*

Gerstenberg, D. L., Osborne, D., & Furlow, W. L. (1979). Inflatable penile prosthesis: follow-up study of patient-partner satisfaction. *Urology, 14,* 583–587.

Gerstenberg, T. C., Metz, P., Ottesen, B., & Fahrenkrug, J. (1991). Intracavernous injection of vasoactive intestinal polypeptide (VIP) and phentolamine in the management of erectile failure. *Journal of Urology, 145,* 404A.

Ginestié, J-F., & Romieu, A. (1976). *L'éxploration radiologique de l'impuissance.* Paris: Maloine.

Giraldi, A., & Wagner, G. (1990). Effect of pinacidil upon penile erectile tissue, in vitro and in vivo. *Pharmacology & Toxicology, 67,* 235–8.

Goldie, L., Kiely, & Williams, G. (1987). Assessment of the immediate and long-term effects of pharmacologically induced penile erections in the treatment of psychogenic and organic impotence. *British Journal of Urology, 59.*

Hedlund, H., & Andersson, K-E. (1985). Contraction and relaxation induced by some prostanoids in isolated human penile erectile tissue and cavernous artery. *Journal of Urology, 134,* 1245–1250.

Holmquist, F., Andersson, K-E., & Hedlund, H. (1990). Effects of pinacidil on isolated human corpus cavernosum penis. *Acta Physiologica Scandinavia, 138,* 463–469.

International Journal of Impotence Research, Suppl. 2, 1990, 1–499.

Ishii, N., Watanabe, H., Irisawa, M., Kikuchi, Y., Kawamura, S., Suzuki, K., Chiba, R., Tokiwa, M., & Shirai, M. (1986). Studies on male sexual impotence. Report 18. Therapeutic trial with prostaglandin E1 for organic impotence. *Japanese Journal of Urology, 77,* 954–957.

Jünemann, et al. (1991). Review of therapy: Pharmacology surgery, methods in Clin Urodyn [special volume]. *Dantec,* 24–27.

Jünemann, K. P., & Alken, P. (1989). Pharmacotherapy of erectile dysfunction. *International Journal of Impotence Research, 1,* 71–93.

Jünemann, K. P., Lue, T. F., Fournier Jr., G. R., & Tanagho, E. A. (1986). Hemodynamics of papaverine- and phentolamine-induced penile erection. *Journal of Urology, 136,* 158–161.

Kaplan, H. S. (1974a). *The New Sex Therapy.* New York: Brunner/Mazel.

Kaplan, H. S. (Winter, 1974b). A new classification of the female sexual dysfunctions. *Journal of Sex & Marital Therapy, 1* (2).

Kaplan, H. S. (Spring, 1977). Hypoactive sexual desire. *Journal of Sex and Marital Therapy, 3* (1).

Kaplan, H. S. (1979). *Disorders of Sexual Desire.* New York: Brunner/Mazel.

Kaplan, H. S. (1980). An integrated approach to brief therapy. In J. Marmor & S. M. Woods (Eds.), *The Interface Between the Psychodynamic and Behavioral Therapies.* New York: Plenum.

Kaplan, H. S. (1983). *The Evaluation of Sexual Disorders: Psychological and Medical Aspects.* New York: Brunner/Mazel.

Kaplan, H. S. (July, 1986). Sexual Problems of the Elderly. Editorial, *American Women's Medical Journal.*

Kaplan, H. S. (with a chapter by Klein, D. F.) (1987). *Sexual Aversion, Sexual Phobias and Panic Disorder.* New York: Brunner/Mazel.

Kaplan, H. S. (1989a). *PE: How to Overcome Premature Ejaculation.* New York: Brunner/Mazel.

Kaplan, H. S. (1989b). The concept of presbyrectia: *International Journal of Impotence Research, 1.*

Kaplan, H. S. (Spring, 1990a). Sex, intimacy and the aging process: *Journal American Academy Psychoanalysis, 18* (1).

Kaplan, H. S. (1990b). Update: Psychogenic impotence. In C. W. Bardin & B. C. Decker (Eds.), *Current Therapy of Endocrinology and Metabolism.* (4th ed.). Philadelphia.

Kaplan, H. S. (Winter, 1990c). The combined use of sex therapy and intrapenil injections in the treatment of impotence. *Journal of Sex & Marital Therapy, 16* (4).

Kaplan, H. S. (1991). Sex therapy with older patients. In W. A. Myers (Ed.), *New Techniques in the Psychotherapy of Older Patients.* Washington, DC: APA Press.

Kaplan, H. S., Freyer, A. J., & Novick, A., (Spring, 1982). The treatment of sexual phobias: The combined use of anti-panic medication and sex therapy. *Journal of Sex & Marital Therapy, 8* (1).

Kinsey, A. C., Pomeroy, W. B., & Martin, C. E. (1953). *Sexual Behavior in the Human Female.* Philadelphia: W. B. Saunders.

Kinsey, A. C., Pomeroy, W. B., Martin, C. E., & Gebhard, P. H. (1948). *Sexual Behavior in the Human Male.* Philadelphia: W. B. Saunders.

Kirkeby, H. J., Anderson, A. J., & Poulsen, E. U. (1989). Nocturnal penile tumescence and rigidity. Translation of data obtained from normal males. *International Journal of Impotence Research, 1,* 115–125.

Klein, D. F. (1987). Sexual disorders and medications. In H. S. Kaplan, *Sexual Aversion, Sexual Phobias and Panic Disorder.* New York: Brunner/Mazel.

Krane, R. J. (1988). Penile prostheses. *Urologic Clinics of North America, 15,* 103–109.

LeFleur, R. S., & Zorgniotti, A. W. (1987). Auto-injection of the corpus cavernosum with a vasoactive drug combination for vasculogenic impotence. *Journal of Urology, 133.*

Leriche, R. (1940). De la résection du carrefour aortoiliaque avec double sympathectomie lombaire pour thrombose arteritique de l'aorte. Le syndrome de lóbliteration terminoaortique par arterie. *Press Medical, 48,* 601–604.

Levine, F. J., & Goldstein, I. (1990). Vascular reconstructive surgery in the management of erectile dysfunction. *International Journal of Impotence Research, 2,* 59–78.

Lue, T. F. (1988). Treatment of venogenic impotence. In E. A. Tanagho, T. F. Lue & R. D. McClure (Eds.), *Contemporary Management of Impotence and Infertility* (pp. 175–177). Baltimore: William & Wilkins.

Lue, T. F., Hricak, H., Marich, K. W., & Tanagho, E. A. (1985). Vasculogenic impotence evaluated by high resolution ultrasonography and pulsed Doppler analysis. *Radiology, 155,* 777–781.

Lue, T. F., Hricak, H., Schmidt, R. A., & Tanagho, E. A. (1986). Functional evaluation of penile veins by cavernosography in papaverine-induced erection. *Journal of Urology, 135,* 479–483.

Lue, T., & Tanagho, E. (1987). Physiology of erection and pharmacological management of impotence. *Journal of Urology, 137.*

Masters, W. B., & Johnson, V. E. (1966). *The Human Sexual Response.* Boston: Little, Brown, & Co.

Masters, W. B., & Johnson, V. E. (1970). *Human Sexual Inadequacy.* Boston: Little, Brown, & Co.

McEwen, B. S., Davis, P. G., & Parson, B. (1979). the brain as a target for steroid hormone action. *Annual Review of Neurosciences, 2,* 65–112.

McMahon, C. G. (1992). The return of potency after intracavernous self injection therapy, personal communication.

Meuleman, E. J. H., Bemelmans, B. L. H., Van Asten, W. N. S. C., Doesburg, W. H., Skotnicki, S. H., & Debruyne, F. M. J. (1990). The value of combined pharmaco-testing and duplex scanning in men with erectile dysfunction. *International Journal of Impotence Research, 2,* 87–98.

Meuleman, E. J. H., Naudin Ten Cate, L., De Wilde, P. C. M., Vooys, G. P., & Debruyne, F. M. J. (1990). The use of penile biopsies in the detection of end-organ disease: a histomorphometric study of the human cavernous body. *International Journal of Impotence Research, 2,* 161–166.

Michal, V., Kramár, R., Pospichal, J., & Hejhal, L. (1973). Direct arterial anastomosis to the cavernous body in the treatment of erectile impotence. *Rozhledy V. Chirugii, 52,* 587–590.

Nadig, P. W. (1989). Six years experience with the vacuum constriction device. *International Journal of Impotence Research, 1,* 55–58.

Newman, H. F. (1970). Vibratory sensitivity of the penis. *Fertility & Sterility, 21,* 791–793.

O'Gorman, E. C., & Bownes, I. T. (1990). Intracavernosal injection therapy for erectile impotence: Ethical, moral and forensic aspects of treatment. *International Journal of Impotence Research, 2,* 99–104.

Ottesen, B., Wagner, G., Virag, R., & Fahrenkrug, J. (1984). Penile erection: Possible role for vasoactive intestinal polypeptide as a neurotransmitter. *British Medical Journal, 288,* 9–11.

Palmore, E. (Ed.). (1970). *Normal Aging*. Durham, NC: Duke University Press.

Palmore, E. (Ed.). (1974). *Normal Aging II*. Durham, NC: Duke University.

Pedersen, B., Tieder, L., Ruiz, M., & Melman, A. (1988). Evaluation of patients and partners 1 to 4 years after penile prosthesis surgery. *Journal of Urology, 139*, 956–958.

Porst, H., & van Ahlen, H. (1989). Pharmakon-induzierte Priapismen—ein Erfahrungsbericht über 101 Falle. *Urologe, 28*, 84–87.

Rajfer, J., Aronson, W. J., Bush, P. A., Frederick, B. S., Dorey, F. J., & Ignarro, L. J. (1992). Nitric oxide as a mediator of relaxation of the corpus cavernosum in response to nonadrenergic, noncholinergic neurotransmission. *New England Journal of Medicine, 326*, 90–94.

Saenz de Tejada, I., Carson, M. P., Traish, A., Eatman, E. H., & Goldstein, I. (1989). Role of endothelin, a novel vasoconstrictor peptide in the local control of penile smooth muscle. *Journal of Urology, 141*, 222A.

Schiavi, R. C., & White, D. (1976). Androgens and male sexual functioning: A review of human studies. *Journal of Sex and Marital Therapy, 2*, 214–228.

Schwartz, A. N., Wang, K. Y., Mack, L. A., Lowe, M., Berger, R. E., Cyr, D. R., & Feldman, M. (1989). Evaluation of normal erectile function with color flow Doppler sonography. *American Journal of Roentgenology, 153*, 1155–1160.

Seagraves, R. T. (1988). Drugs and desire. In R. S. Leiblum & R. C. Rosen (Eds.), *Sexual Desire Disorders*. New York: Guilford.

Seagraves, R. T. (1988). Hormones and libido. In S. R. Leiblum & R. C. Rosen (Eds.), *Sexual Desire Disorders*. New York: Guilford.

Seagraves, R.T., & Seagraves, K. B. (1992). Aging and drug effects on amle sexuality. In R. C. Rosen & S. R. Leiblum (Eds.), *Erectile Disorders: Assessment and Treatment*. New York: Guilford.

Seamans, J. H. (1956). Premature ejaculation: A new approach. *Southern Urological Journal, 49*.

Sjöstrand, N. O., & Klinge, E. (1979). Principal mechanisms controlling penile retraction and protrusion in rabbits. *Acta Physiologica Scandinavia, 106*, 199–207.

Stackl, W., Hasun, R., & Marberger, M. (1988). Intracavernous injection of prostaglandin E_1 in impotent men. *Journal of Urology, 140*, 66–68.

Starr, B. D., & Weiner, M. B. (1981). *The Starr-Weiner Report on Sex and Sexuality in the Mature Years*. New York: McGraw-Hill.

Steiness, I. (1957). Vibratory perception in normal subjects. *Acta Medica Scandinavica, 158,* 315–327.

Stief, C. G., Bernard, F., Bosch, R. J. L. H., Aboseif, S. R., Lue, T., & Tanagho, E. (1990). A possible role for calcitonin-gene-related peptide in the regulation of the smooth muscle tone of the bladder and penis. *Journal of Urology, 143,* 392–397.

Todarello, O., & Boscia, F. M. (1985). Sexuality in aging: A study of a group of 300 elderly men and women. *Journal of Endocrinological Investigation, 8,* (suppl. 2).

Tudoriu, T., & Bourmer, H. (1983). The hemodynamics of erection at the level of the penis and its local deterioration. *Journal of Urology, 129,* 741–745.

Turner, A. L., Althof, E. D., Levine, S. B., Risen, C. B., Bocheer, D. R., Kursh, E. D. Bocheer, & Resnick, M. I. (Fall, 1989). Self-injection of papaverine and phentolamine in the treatment of psychogenic impotence. *Journal of Sex and Marital Therapy, 15* (3).

Virag, R. (1982). Intracavernous injection of papaverine for erectile failure. *Lancet, 2,* 938.

Virag, R. (et al.) (1985). Is impotence an arterial disease? A study of arterial risk factors in 440 impotent men. *Lancet, I,* 181–184.

Wagner, G. (1985). Penile erection provoked by vibration and intracorporal injection. *Nordisk Sexologi, 3,* 113–119.

Wagner, G. (1986). The influence of oestrogen on vaginal physiology—Symptomatology of oestrogen deprived women. In P. B. Eriksen & G. Samsiol (Eds.), *The Urogenital Oestrogen Deficiency Syndrome.* Proceedings of International Workshop. Copenhagen: Nov. 7.

Wagner, G. (1991). In U. Jonas et al. (Eds.), *Erectile Dysfunction: Neuropharmacology of penile erection in vitro* (pp. 57–58). Berlin, Heidelberg: Springer-Verlag.

Wagner, G., & Brindley, G. S. (1980). The effect of atropine, α and β blockers on human penile erection: A controlled pilot study. In A. W. Zorgniotti & G. Rossi (Eds.), Vasculogenic Impotence: *Proceedings of 1st International Conference on Corpus Cavernosum Revascularization* (pp. 77–81). Springfield, IL: Charles C Thomas.

Wagner, G., & Gerstenberg, T. (1987). Intracavernosal injection of vasoactive intestinal polypeptide (VIP) does not induce erection in man per se. *World Journal of Urology, 5,* 171–177.

Wagner, G., & Green, R. (1981). *Impotence: Physiological, Psychological, Surgical Diagnosis and Treatment.* New York: Plenum Press.

Watters, G. R., Keogh, E. J., Earle, C. M., Carati, C. J., Wisiewski, Z. S.,

Tulloch, A. G. & Lord, D. J. (1988). Experience in the management of erectile dysfunction using the intercavernosal self-injection of vasoactive drugs. *Journal of Urology, 140*.

Wein, A. J., Arsdalen, K. V., & Levin, R. M. (1983). Adrenergic corporal receptors. In R. J. Krane, H. B. Siroky & I. Goldstein (Eds.), *Male Sexual Function* (pp. 33–37). Boston: Little, Brown.

Weiss, A. D. (1971). Sensory functions. In J. E. Birren (Ed.), *Handbook of Aging and the Individual.* Chicago: University of Chicago Press.

Weitzman, R., & Hart, J. (1987). Sexual behavior in healthy, elderly married men. *Archives of Sexual Behavior, 16*.

Willis, E., Ottesen, B., Fahrenkrug, J., Sundler, F., & Wagner, G. (1981). Vasoactive intestinal polypeptide as a possible neurotransmitter in penile erection. *Acta Physiologica Scandinavia, 113*, 545–546.

Zorgniotti, A. W., & Lefleur, R. S. (1985). Auto-injection of the corpus cavernosum with a vasoactive drug combination for vasculogenic impotence. *Journal of Urology, 133*, 39–41.

Zorgniotti, A. W., & Lizza, E. F. (1991). *Diagnosis and Management of Impotence.* Philadelphia: Decker.

Index